CANCER WARRIOR
Where the Mind Goes

Ruth Levine

Quill House Publishers
Minneapolis, Minnesota

CANCER WARRIOR
Where the Mind Goes
Ruth Levine

The author, out of traditional Jewish respect for reference to the Almighty in secular print, uses the term "G-d" instead of writing out the word in full.

ISBN - 13: 978-1-933794-41-9
ISBN - 10: 1-933794-41-0
LCCN: 2011922881

Quill House Publishers, PO Box 390759, Minneapolis, MN 55439
Manufactured in the United States of America

Table of Contents

To the memory of Dr. Michael Stark
and Dr. W. Douglas Wong
who were a better kind of cancer warrior

Prologue

"Ruth, wake up."

An unfamiliar voice was nudging me awake, prying me from a deep, comforting sleep – the type of sleep which enfolds you like a downy blanket on a rainy winter night. But it was a mid-morning in early August, and my deep sleep had not been induced by rain but by anesthesia. It was comforting nonetheless.

"Wake up, Ruth. It's time to wake up."

I breathed shallowly, but without effort or discomfort. The thin tubing of a nasal canula brought a cool, gentle stream of oxygen into my nostrils. But there was no breathing tube jammed down my throat. No breathing tube! So, they were true to their word. What a joy to wake up without it! My eyes opened into sleepy slits then closed again. A thought entered my drowsy head, and I raised my hand to touch my stomach just below and to the right of my belly button.

"It's gone. You have a dressing there now. Don't touch it."

I slid my hand down to my side and opened my eyes to bright florescent surroundings. The recovery room didn't look dark and shadowy as it had the first time around. That had been way different from this.

But, let me backtrack, because I have a story to tell you, and I need to tell it from the beginning. A lot of people have told me that I should write it down. So, as I begin the next phase of my life, I think it would be a good idea to follow their advice. I'm big on following good advice. And, I believe it's partly due to the fact that I follow such advice that I'm still here to tell you all about it. By now you must be thinking that I'm a bit self absorbed to presume that I have a message within me that's worthwhile recording. I'll admit it – I am. But if you had lived through what I have, you too would probably feel that there is a Higher Power directing events and guiding you through, so that some greater good might be reached in the end. And if I can help even one other person, then what does it matter if it's my ego which is driving me on? Possibly my story will help you get through a huge challenge. Maybe it will teach you things that you can take with you and use in the face of a daunting circumstance. It's a story of grave illness, despair, belief, hope, and mental resolve. It's my epic tale – my own odyssey – one which involves many of life's profound experiences. And it began in the middle of my ordinary life, at the beginning of my fiftieth year.

First, let me tell you a bit about myself. Mike, my husband, and I have been married now for twenty-six years. We live in a simple townhouse in a Jersey suburb and have two kids – a twenty-year-old son, Zack, and a sixteen-year-old daughter, Lia. We are two people who have each changed careers in mid-life. About eight years ago, Mike sold his chiropractic practice and entered the teaching field. During his transition, he went back to school in the evenings and acquired certification in special education, school counseling, and substance abuse counseling. He's now a high school guidance counselor and has recently earned his master's degree in that field.

As for me, five years ago I left my job as a special education aide and entered an occupational therapy master's program at a state university. For a long time I had wanted to enter a profession where I could help children in a very direct way. After observing occupational therapists where I worked, I felt that was the field for me. So, I left my comfortable niche and set out in a new direction, going to school at night at a nearby community college for the necessary prerequisite classes. I was driven, got straight A's, and was then accepted into the full-time OT program.

Some might say that the career moves which Mike and I have made in mid-life are remarkable. But a lot of people do stuff like that. You have to be totally focused on it and want it more than anything. My focus on my own goal was laser sharp, so sharp that I pushed aside everything else to concentrate on completing the OT program. Everything – husband, friends, kids, and home – became secondary to the primary goal of getting my degree. It was a challenging curriculum, and some aspects of it, such as the research project and my physical disabilities fieldwork, were especially so for me. But I got through them, although I did take a four-month break to decompress from all the stress. Then, in the fall of 2005, there only remained my pediatric fieldwork and the national exam to take. And that's where my story really begins.

Silently Within

In many ways, Walton School in suburban Springfield, where I did my pediatric affiliation, was idyllic. The staff there made it so. For the most part, there was a feeling of camaraderie and teamwork in this elementary school. And my supervisor, Jan, was great, as she always was on hand to observe and give me constructive criticism in a very non-threatening way. But the commute was a bitch and the weekly preparation, paperwork and eventually, case study, adaptive equipment project, and, of course, the evaluations, felt endless. My Saturdays were spent studying for the boards. Saturday nights and Sundays were for preparing activities. Weekday evenings were for paperwork. But, after having had a bad experience during my previous physical disabilities fieldwork, I was determined to do well in this one. I threw all my effort into my work and blocked out everything and everyone else.

The only sore spot in my experience at Walton School was a nagging stomach virus which I had caught. It had been raging among the students. Now, in mid-October, I had it. Every weekday morning, despite a feeling of not having quite emptied my bowels, I would get into my car and make the long commute north, my stomach churning. It got to a point where, in order to counteract the feeling of having to go frequently to the bathroom, I was eating only binding foods such as bagels and pretzels for lunch. As the fall term progressed, my bowel movements appeared narrower and lighter in color than usual. Attributing it to stress, I made a mental note to call my internist, Dr. Stark, when fieldwork was all done, to have myself checked out. Back in September I was supposed to have had my first routine colonoscopy, but had postponed it to avoid conflict with my fieldwork schedule. I told myself that I would reschedule that, too.

"You probably have a spastic ilium or some colitis."

That was Mike's impression as he adjusted me on the portable chiropractic adjusting table in our living room. It was late December. Fieldwork had thankfully ended, and I now had ten days to study in earnest for the boards, which were scheduled for January 2. That was the last day to take the test in the allotted three-month window of time which I was given after registering for the exam. Now, with the immediate pressure of fieldwork gone, I could allow some time for Mike to adjust me.

"Maybe it's just nerves and it'll clear up after I take the exam."

I truly believed this. But for now, I would spend ten days totally focused on reabsorbing information which I had learned in school in preparation for the big test. I realized that I really had not been focusing on studying during fieldwork, for I was doing very poorly on the computerized practice exams which I took at home. And, ideally, I should have given myself about three months after fieldwork had ended to prepare, as I knew some people had done. Oh, well. After making a study schedule, I put in eight to ten hours a day to go through my review book. I'm fortunate that I'm able to totally focus on a subject – provided I make up my mind to do so! Well, my mind was made up. The exam, which would determine whether I would become a certified occupational therapist, was less than ten days away. To the virtual exclusion of everything else, I plowed into my studies.

By the time January 2 came around, I was experiencing intermittent pain in the right upper quadrant of my abdomen. So, before leaving for the exam, I took two Ibuprofen tablets, to take the edge off. I felt well prepared for the test and was confident that I would pass. Nevertheless, I spent the entire four-hour time allotment carefully contemplating the 200 questions and returning to the ones of which I was not sure. As I became totally engrossed in the exam, I completely forgot the pain in my right side.

That evening, my stomach symptoms seemed to let up. They surely must have been the result of the unrelenting mental pressure which I had been under for the past four months. Everyone knows that the mind can do funny things to the body. And I would have skipped going to Dr. Stark if my symptoms had not returned the next day. So I made my appointment with him, and with my gynecologist as well, to rule out any problems in that area.

"It could be your gall bladder."

Dr. Stark was listening to my chest through his stethoscope. He seemed concerned. He had given me a clean bill of health only four and a half months earlier during my yearly checkup. Could he have missed something then? My blood pressure was also a little high now.

"Well, that's because you're not feeling well," said Dr. Stark, as he held my wrist to feel for my pulse.

How do you like that? I turn fifty, and my body parts start to go. Remembering the pain and discomfort that a neighbor had endured after her gall bladder was removed, I silently contemplated the aftermath of such a surgery. Dr. Stark gave me a script for an ultrasound of my gall bladder and arranged for me to meet in two days with Dr. C, a gastroenterologist who worked out of his office once a week. How convenient for me, I noted, not without a touch of sarcasm. Dr. Stark assured me that Dr. C was quite competent. I left his office feeling for the first time in my life not like a person but like a patient – someone whose health is off kilter and on whom tests and procedures are endlessly performed. It was a crappy, uneasy feeling.

"What the hell . . . ?"

Two days later, Dr. Barth, my gynecologist, was giving me a pelvic exam. It felt as if he had half his arm up inside of me, and he looked concerned. Seven months earlier I had been to him for my yearly check up, and everything had been fine then. I started to hyperventilate from the pressure of his arm.

"Easy, easy."

Dr. Barth always knew how to calm me, but it was apparent that he felt something strange, something hard. After I got dressed, he wrote me a script for a pelvic ultrasound "to get to the bottom of this." I wasn't too concerned yet. After all, perhaps I had a big fibroid? That was a common thing at my age. Little did I know that a relentless barrage of medical testing was about to begin.

The ultrasound of my gall bladder showed nothing on that organ. But when I went to Dr. Stark's office to pick up a copy of the report, he was waiting there to speak with me.

"The gall bladder is clear, but something has shown up on your liver."

That "something," he said, was humongous – seven inches in length, took up most of the right lobe, and, according to the report, could possibly indicate a "primary or metastatic neoplasm" – cancer.

"They have to cover themselves by writing that, don't they?" I asked naively.

I really believed that. Dr. Stark then took my hand into both of his and gently explained that a colleague of his had also had a large "mass" on his liver, and that he was now fine. I went numb. Then I felt panic pulse through my body. I decided not to look at the report until I got home. It wouldn't be good to freak out while driving.

"I need to talk to you," I quietly told Mike shortly after he arrived home that day. It seemed like I had waited ages for him. His expression froze as he immediately sensed the seriousness in my voice. After Lia had gone upstairs, I related what had happened and showed him the report. He slowly sat down next to me at the kitchen table, taking it all in. The enormity of the situation was engulfing me, bringing me to a very bleak place in my mind – an abyss, down which lay the dark face of death. I could scarcely speak. My words came out slow and stammering.

"I suppose at worst, death is just a blankness, and I shouldn't be afraid of that. But," I continued between suppressed sobs, "I . . . don't . . . want . . . to leave." The thought of leaving this earth and my family behind overwhelmed me. And then I cried in his arms.

But one diagnostic test is not definitive. The pelvic ultrasound which Dr. Barth prescribed showed that I had some sort of pelvic mass. A program which I had watched on the Discovery Channel had documented the case of an older woman who was carrying the mummified remains of her unborn fetus, around which was growing a large tumor. Perhaps I had one of those? I was grasping at any possibility. Anything but cancer. As far as the liver mass was concerned, Dr. Barth said that it could even be a hemangioma – a large, benign, tangled mass of blood vessels, which about thirty percent of all women have, and that I shouldn't jump to any conclusions. So I calmed down a bit. As a matter of fact, the next test ordered by Dr. Stark – a CAT scan of my chest, abdomen, and pelvis – suggested that the large mass on my liver was indeed a hemangioma. That was a relief. But could it be removed? The CAT scan also showed a lesion in my pelvic area, and the radiologist recommended that I follow up with a pelvic MRI and a nuclear blood pool study of my liver to clarify what these things really were.

Meanwhile, the pain in my right side was already slowing me down. Walking fast had been my sole form of exercise, and the pain was now interfering with that. Furthermore, I was now beginning to feel a strange, dull ache in my right shoulder. After some investigation on the Internet, I learned that liver tumors can cause this referred pain because of a nerve which runs from the liver up to the shoulder. So, I called Dr. Stark to tell him my opinion that this mass was indeed a tumor. He agreed that I was probably right.

Like gathering storm clouds, the pain which was now taking hold of me brought with it a vague feeling of dread as I went about my days. Something dark and threatening, but as yet unnamed, was slowly, relentlessly taking shape, entwining itself into the fabric of my life. However, Dr. Stark was also relentless in ordering test after test to identify those storm clouds, and wasting no time, I faithfully made one appointment after another to get those tests done. That's how it was in January 2006.

Four days after the CAT scan, Mike took me for my colonoscopy, performed by Dr. C at a local gastrointestinal diagnostic center. Let me tell you, the worst part of a colonoscopy is the prep – anyone who's had one will attest to that. The exam itself is easy, for you are put under anesthesia. After the procedure, I woke up in a recovery bed, feeling completely relaxed, as if I had the most wonderful sleep. After getting dressed, Mike and I waited in a consultation room to discuss the results with Dr. C.

My feeling of complete relaxation was not to last. When she came into the consultation room, the first words out of Dr. C's mouth were, "I'm afraid I have some bad news." These unfortunate words seemed to reverberate in the air and bored deeply into me, creating a well of alarm.

Then she continued.

"You have a rather large tumor in your rectum. It's circumferential, and I had to use a narrower scope to get past it to examine your colon."

I could feel the adrenaline rushing through me, spreading panic. And I immediately felt that Dr. C's way of delivering this news was unprofessional, in that it only served to induce that panic. Immediately, I made a quick mental note to eliminate her from my treatment team should I turn out to be sick. Then my mind took a different turn. A tumor, I thought, is not necessarily malignant. A biopsy had been taken, and the pathology results would tell what this tumor really was. Until then, I would hold onto this shard of hope.

But I was of two minds. On the one hand, nothing was absolutely certain yet, and I held onto the hope that all would turn out well. On the other hand, Dr. C's opening remarks in the consultation room set the stage for a downward spiral, for the next day I noticed a dull pain in my rectum. My legs were achy, and I just didn't feel like eating. My stools were frequent, narrow, and bloody – probably from the biopsy. A few days after the colonoscopy, I realized that I had begun to run a daily fever in the afternoons. Perhaps it was psychosomatic, but I also had trouble taking a deep breath.

In addition to showing the "mass" in my rectum, the pelvic MRI which I had taken also indicated a prominent lymph node. This new finding wasn't at all alarming to me, because in my naiveté I did not equate this with a malignancy. But then I went for the nuclear blood pool scan of my liver. As I lay on the table within the huge donut-shaped contraption, I mused about how I was getting radiated up the wazoo. In the course of only a few weeks, I had enough radiation to last a lifetime. After being injected with a radioactive dye, it took at least another forty-five minutes for the administration of this test; I lay on my back with my arms crossed above the crown of my head, and spent the time talking with the technician about the surgery she had for her varicose veins. Then she got very quiet as she observed the scans of my liver on the monitor. When it was finally over and I got up from the table to leave, she gave me a look of horror which one reserves for the doomed. Her look disturbed me. Emotions are contagious and although I wasn't quite sure if she was overreacting, that horrified feeling crossed the space between us and entered into me. When I received the radiologist's report a few days later, I knew why the technician had looked at me that way. The liver lesion – a huge thing, all in the right lobe – appeared to be a neoplasm. Cancer.

Thank G-d for Debbie. She's my good friend who is completely logical and compassionate. "Whenever you need to talk to me, just call, even if it's in the middle of the night. I'll be there for you," she had told me. Though I now hardly slept at night, I couldn't bring myself to disturb her at all hours. Instead, I took her advice to listen to the radio next to my bed when I couldn't go back to sleep. I did that a lot.

I was in the bathroom. Frequent bowel movements were now typical for me. The telephone rang. I heard Dr. C's urgent voice on the answering machine, telling me to call her back immediately. Breathless, I rushed out of the bathroom and picked up the phone before she hung up.

"Your rectal tumor is malignant," she said. She sounded panicky herself. "And, it's a very aggressive form of cancer. You need to take care of this immediately."

Alarm and despair surged through me like a tidal wave. Mike had already spoken to people about oncologists, and several had recommended Dr. Nissenblatt. He was a well-established doctor, but unfortunately, was not taking on any new patients. However, he had several associates, and we had made an appointment with one of them – Dr. Salwitz – just in case my tumor was malignant. Struggling now to think rationally, I asked Dr. C to call Salwitz to see if she could move up my appointment with him.

As I sat next to Mike that evening on the couch, I opened up.

"Mike, I think I may need some anti-anxiety medication."

Previously, I would have looked upon such meds as a terrible crutch – a foreign thing which I never would have used. But now I was engulfed by an overwhelming anxiety which I just couldn't seem to get a handle on, no matter with whom I spoke. Mike understood.

"Maybe you should try Reiki. I could get in touch with Paulette."

Mike had gone to weekly Reiki sessions a year and a half earlier. I had never gone with him or to them, quietly scoffing at the notion that anything positive could result from this "light touch therapy." But now I was vulnerable and needy, and was willing to try anything. I asked him to make an appointment with Paulette. Mike also got in touch with Memorial Sloan Kettering. After I faxed them copies of my radiology reports and arranged for the biopsy slides to be sent to them, they booked us to see Dr. Wong, Chief of Colorectal Surgery. At the same time, in order to get another perspective, I made an appointment with a local colorectal surgeon, Dr. Z, who had success-fully operated on Debbie's neighbor a few years back.

"How are you today?"

That was the standard, now outrageous question which every checkout clerk was trained to ask each customer.

"How the hell do you think I am? I have cancer!"

That's what I wanted to snap at them. But I restrained myself. They couldn't help that they didn't know. How could anyone know, just by looking at me, that cancer was silently taking hold?

Lost in a fearful fog, I went about my days barely able to focus on the simplest tasks. Once, when turning a corner in my car, I was so distracted by my anxiety that I drove too close to the curb and punc-tured a tire. A kind stranger, or should I say angel, stopped his car and offered to change the flat. And so it would be in the coming months. I would not be alone. There would always be people coming into my life who would help and guide me along the dark road. And always there was Mike, who harnessed his own anxiety into action, so that we could confront the cancer in the best possible way.

Never having faced death before, I now had a life-threatening illness and I felt as though I was standing at the edge of a very deep abyss. Although I have always believed in G-d, I hadn't prayed to him in a personal, meaningful way in a very long time – certainly not since beginning the occupational therapy program three and a half years before. But I now felt a primal need to reconnect to the Almighty and to plead to him to spare me. The evening after Dr. C called, I waited until everyone had gone up to bed. Feeling a despondency which I had never experienced before, I took out my father's talis bag which I kept in a cabinet in the living room. Unfolding the deep creases of the yellowing prayer shawl, I flung it over my head and enwrapped my-self in its folds. Women do not pray while wearing men's prayer shawls, but this was no ordinary prayer. I didn't read from a prayer book, nor did I speak, for my wracking sobs left no room for words in my throat.

Now it was time to tell my other friends and relatives. All were supportive. Risa, however, actually wailed over the phone.

"It's not fair!" she cried when I told her about my rectal and liver tumors. She started to bawl hysterically.

"Stop it!" I ordered. "I'm through with that!"

I was vehement. Although riddled with anxiety, I had now moved past the sobbing stage, and I needed my friends to be strong and supportive. Tears and pity would only drag me down more into that dark place. I was prepared to sever all contact with anyone – friend or relative – who could not be totally positive. Risa then calmed down and told me about her cousin, who had stomach cancer, which is nearly always fatal. He became very religious and went into spontaneous remission. I needed to hear things like that. It was the first story of hope which I had heard, and as I was to learn, hearing the success stories of others was just as empowering to me emotionally as it must have been to those who had actually lived through them.

Everyone asked if they could help me – if I needed anything. No, I was still functional. But I had absolutely no appetite. Healthy people have appetites. Those on a downward spiral have little need for nutrition, for death requires no sustenance. I ate what little I could, not out of hunger, but because I knew that is what people are supposed to do in order to live. What I needed most was prayer. So, I told everyone who asked that what I needed them to do was to pray for me – not to just think a good thought, but to actually move their lips and pray, either formally or informally, either at home or in church or synagogue, and to do it with complete concentration. What I needed was an army of people petitioning G-d on my behalf. For this was war – I felt like a body under siege – and at the beginning, prayer was my sole weapon. My friend Barbara insisted that I pray formally every day – at least every morning and evening – even if I only did an abridged version of the lengthy prayers. And so I began to pray, both from a prayer book and also off the cuff. Just meet me halfway – that's all I asked of G-d. Meet me halfway, and I will do the rest.

That Saturday morning, Mike and I went to synagogue, something I used to do regularly before going back to school. We both felt the need to pray within a group. It is often said in orthodox circles that a group context potentiates prayer. That is why observant Jews pray in a quorum. During a lull in the services, after coming out of the bathroom, I ran into the Rabbi in the hallway. He greeted me enthusiastically and asked how I was and if I had finished the OT program. I gave him the latest news. He stood there with his mouth opened. He was floored.

"That's terrible news! I'm so sorry! If there's anything we can do, don't hesitate to ask. We'll certainly add your name to the list of people receiving a '*meshebarach*' (i.e., a get well prayer). Have you started treatment? You know, nowadays there are many wonderful new therapies. It's not like it was years ago. What a terrible thing to happen to you just as you've finished your studies!"

He was sympathetic – yes. But I felt there was one important element missing from his response. I could always find out about new therapies from doctors, friends, and from the Internet. My ears were hanging onto each word he said, anticipating some spiritual message. The Rabbi proceeded to give practical advice. I interrupted him.

"Rabbi," I said definitively, "it's G-d's will."

He stopped and stared at me. These were the words which I needed to hear from him – these words and more. Somewhat disappointed, I must admit, I returned to my seat in the sanctuary. Since then, I've learned that it is considered callous to tell a very ill person, "It's G-d's will," for they may take that as a very flippant, uncaring remark, and they may actually respond better to practical suggestions. However, I'm not like that, and I wanted nothing more than to delve into the deeper meaning of my illness.

Although the Rabbi did not focus on the spiritual, we are blessed with many ancient sages whose wise, comforting words have come down to us through the generations. One of them was Rabbi Akiva, who, among other things, was noted for always saying, "Whatever G-d does is for my good." Throughout my entire journey into illness, I repeated these words in my mind, over and over, until they penetrated and until I believed them utterly.

It was a cold, gray afternoon in early February when Mike and I first went to the clinic in East Brunswick to see Dr. Salwitz. We sat anxiously in the spacious, modern waiting room and read psalms. Finally, we were called into the lab where they took a blood sample. After my vitals were taken, we were ushered into the examination room. A nurse practitioner, who introduced herself as Janice, came in and took down my history. She was very compassionate. But more important than this, she was positive – telling me that I was young, that aside from the cancer, I was basically in good health, and that she believed I would do well. I was convinced that Mike and I had come to the right place.

After a short wait, Dr. Salwitz entered. He had been studying my reports and films.

"Hello, beautiful," he addressed me.

My face was flushed from the fever I had been running in the afternoons ever since the colonoscopy. Perhaps he meant that I had a nice, pink complexion; I couldn't imagine that he meant it any other way, as I had never considered myself to be physically beautiful. Dr. Salwitz, a quick moving man in a compact body, was upbeat and exuded a nervous energy which I found invigorating.

"Your cancer is treatable," he told us. Mind you, he did not use the word "curable," but treatable sounded pretty good to me.

"The good news is that the liver tumor appears to be confined to the lower right lobe and can be surgically removed."

Dr. Salwitz suggested a course of treatment starting with chemo, to shrink the rectal tumor, followed by colorectal surgery at Robert Wood Johnson University Hospital, a recuperative period of two months, and then liver surgery at another hospital which had a "top" liver surgeon.

"Why can't I have both surgeries done at one shot?" I asked. Why should I have to be cut open twice?

"Because one place is clean and the other one is dirty," was his answer.

I mulled over this rationale. Dr. Salwitz then made sure that the front office arranged for me to have a liver MRI and a full body PET scan to see where any other tumors might be lurking; he mentioned that I would eventually have a mediport placement so that I could begin chemotherapy. Salwitz wasted no time in getting things moving. The initial lab reports came back to him. My blood CEA level, which measures the presence of enzymes given off by cancer cells, was 427. Normal is from 0 to 2.5. My body was infested with cancer cells. If I had my way, I would have dived into a vat of chemo right then and there. It would be another weapon at my disposal, and like a city under siege, I felt that I was holding on desperately until an allied army arrived to help me fight off the enemy.

Now it was time to tell Zack and Lia. They knew that something was wrong with me, but we had delayed telling them what it was until we were absolutely certain. It was now time to be up front.

"Come here," I called to them shortly after we returned from Dr. Salwitz. Mike and I stood together at the bottom of the staircase, our coats still on.

"I have something to tell both of you, and I don't want to have to repeat it." Saying it once would be hard enough.

They both came near, quiet, tense, sensing the importance of the moment.

"We found out what's wrong with me." I took a deep breath. "I have cancer."

A bomb shell.

"Where?" asked Lia.

"It's in my rectum and has spread to my liver."

Another bombshell dropped.

"But," I continued, "we've just been to an oncologist, and he's said that it's treatable."

"Are you going to get chemo?" asked Zack.

"Eventually, yes. And I'll have surgery too, eventually."

Lia, fifteen at the time, was still blessed with some childhood innocence.

"Will you lose your hair?" she asked, for in her limited experience, nothing could be worse than that in what lay ahead.

"I may. We'll see."

So, I handed a bombshell to them with one hand, but balanced it by hope in the other. At least I was able to give them that.

I couldn't keep the conclusive news from my mother any longer. She knew something was very wrong and had even accompanied me to a few of my scans. So, I suppose when I told her that I definitely had cancer, she wasn't totally shocked. She herself had been living with non-Hodgkin's lymphoma for about eleven years.

As was our weekly custom, I went to pick her up by car to take her to the farmer's market. After I broke the bad news, she went about discussing the situation in a very practical way.

"It's from stress, you know."

I nodded. I had read about how stress may play a role in the development of cancer. As I drove, I ticked off for us all of the stressful events which had happened to me over the past two years: my father's death from metastatic liver cancer, which followed the death of my aunt by one day – we had back-to-back funerals; a school research paper which never seemed to be good enough for my professors and which I worked on for two months even after my class had graduated; not going to graduation because I had not yet completed my paper; a stressful physical disabilities fieldwork experience with a supervisor whom I felt neglected his supervisory duties and was hyper-critical on the occasions when he was available; the cutting down of most of the beautiful woods beyond our grassy back yard to make way for a new senior housing development; Zack's arrest for possession of marijuana in his car; the long, congested commute to my last fieldwork; and the nonstop schedule I lived in order to get through it. That would be enough to put anyone over the thin line which separated good health from illness.

"I have something to give you when we get back. You know," my mother went on, "when I was first diagnosed with lymphoma, I was very depressed. But then I read this book, and I told myself, 'The hell with all this!' It was very helpful, and after reading it, I completely changed my attitude and just didn't worry about it anymore."

When we came back to her home, I helped my mother with her packages. In my pain and growing fatigue, I straggled behind as she strode ahead of me up the walkway. Once inside, she retrieved the book from her small living room bookcase: *Fighting Cancer*. It was to be the first of many books I was to read on the subject – the first of many books which focused only on the positive – the first source which told me that cancer was not a death sentence. But, when you have a large malignant tumor on a vital organ, it certainly feels like one.

It was a lovely ride to Long Branch, to Paulette the Reiki master, but exhausting for me, as I was now becoming quite debilitated. By this time, early February, I was no longer able to walk for more than ten minutes at a time, and I was as tired as an old woman. Grocery shopping, even with a car, was a great effort, and I was physically unable to make more than one outing a day. The fever I had been running was now beginning earlier – in mid-morning – and I felt very ill most of the day and all night. Anxiety and a sense of foreboding lay continually upon my heart. On top of this, I was in pain much of the time, experiencing simultaneous dull and sharp pain in my rectum and a sharp pain in my right abdomen where my liver was. This last pain radiated dully up into my right shoulder. What distressed me most was that cooking, even the simplest meals, was now a supreme effort for me, and I no longer felt up to the task. My mother insisted in coming over in the evenings to prepare dinner. Sometimes Gary, my brother, would drive her over, and sometimes it would be Mike. Funny, that at the age of eighty-nine, when she had moved from Florida to be near us in her old age, it was now she who was becoming the caretaker. And who would take care of her, should I soon die? Meanwhile, my mother was still sharp enough to come up with ideas, here and there, to make my life easier.

"You know, my neighbor told me that you could apply for a handicapped license plate." This would allow me to park in handicapped spots. But I didn't want any of the trappings of illness, including special license plates. Nor did I want to take on the persona of a patient. I needed to feel as normal as possible. To her dismay, I refused to apply for the handicapped plates.

So, after getting directions from Paulette, Mike and I drove to Long Branch one Sunday morning in early February. She lived in a very fancy building at the shore. The large, bright, and airy lobby had a subtle, yet pleasing scent which I couldn't quite identify. A hint of this strange scent followed us into the elevator and down the hallway. When she opened the door of her apartment, I was surprised to see an older woman, for Paulette sounded much younger over the telephone. Yet, her hair was nearly all dark, unlike mine, which is now a salt and pepper color, and her facial skin was still rather smooth. Paulette was warm, friendly, and down to earth. Her apartment was decorated in a style which I can only describe as "eclectic oriental," and it was filled with many paintings and sculptures. It was a soothing décor.

We all sat down on the large sectional in the living room.

"Mike, she's beautiful!"

How embarrassing, this sudden, open compliment by this stranger, given as if she were looking at a photo! It was a compliment which always embarrassed me, for I never believed it to be true. I felt myself blush. We then began to talk about my health situation and what we had done and were still to do about it. During our conversation, I silently tried to assess whether I could trust this new person. She took notes on a pad as we spoke.

Paulette then explained to me what Reiki is and what she would be doing. While she sat on a therapy ball, she would be touching, gently, various areas of my body, but mostly my head, for that, she said, was where my anxiety lay. That was fine, I thought, for I had never liked deep massage. Paulette explained that Reiki would help me to achieve a calm state so that I could begin to heal, that the effects of the Reiki were cumulative, and that each Reiki session could feel different. I pondered over what she said. The word "heal" sounded very noncommittal to me. One could heal physically or spiritually. Which way did she mean? And the exact meaning of the word was subject to interpretation. I felt that "heal" was to "remission" as "treat" was to "cure." The word "heal" just didn't go far enough. However, I decided that for me, "healing" would mean a complete physical healing and nothing less.

Mike went into the spare bedroom to read, and Paulette then directed me to lie down supine on the massage table in her living room, with my head on a small pillow. She covered me with a blanket, lit some candles, and talked me through a deep breathing exercise. It was very similar to meditation, in that one focuses on one's breath and clears the mind of all thoughts.

"Do you need more blankets?"

Paulette noticed that I was shivering. It was from the fever I had been running. So she tucked two more blankets around me, and I began to warm up.

As Paulette began to do the actual Reiki, standing at the head of the massage table, she moved her hands in circular motions over her head and around her middle. Suppressing all skepticism, I watched with an open mind. She turned on the CD player, and the strands of a very relaxing, new age musical piece began to play.

"And as we begin," intoned Paulette in a quiet, slow, soothing voice, "try to have a sense of a light – a strong, white, healing light energy entering your body through the top of your head. Every time you breathe in, you're breathing in this light, and when you breathe out, you're releasing everything that does not serve you. Have a sense of this light traveling through you, through your blood, your bones, your nerves, as it enters into every cell of your body and every recess of your mind, giving you peace, comfort, joy, health, and clarity, knowing that it is all for your highest good. So be it."

I then felt Paulette put her hands on the crown of my head – hands which were remarkably warm for an older woman (she was probably old enough to be my mother – although a young mother). Applying my powers of concentration, I visualized in detail a bright, sparkling light which took on the physical consistency of a thin stream of molasses; slowly, slowly it glided along each of my organ systems, from head to toe, finally entering into me on the cellular level. I especially concentrated on this light entering my rectum and liver, as Paulette directed.

"Relax your shoulders. Let them sink into the table." I obeyed.

"Relax your jaw. Let it go slack." Yes ma'am.

"Relax the space between your eyes." I stopped frowning.

"You have your eyes opened. Try closing them." Once again, I did as I was told.

I felt her hands over the part of my body where my liver was. After a while, I opened my eyes. Her hands were hovering a few feet above my abdomen, yet it felt as if they were still lying on me. Now, that was very curious.

"You know," suggested Paulette, "when you're sitting in the clinic getting chemo, it may help you to have a sense of this light energy coming into you."

I looked up at her. I had read about visualization and illness, all right. So many cancer survivors have told of how they imagined, in detail, destroying their tumors.

"When I get chemo," I declared fiercely, "I'm going to visualize slaughtering all the cancer cells with a machete. The chemo will be medieval knights with swords. We're gonna hack the tumors to death. There's going to be a blood bath."

Did she find it shocking that I would have such a violent fantasy? But Paulette sounded approving when she answered, "You're very visual. And you're a warrior."

The Reiki session lasted an hour, after which Mike came out of the adjacent room and stood next to the massage table.

"Well," Paulette asked me, "how was it?"

As if I had just awakened, although I had never been asleep, I sat up on the table, with my legs stretched out before me. Paulette handed me a glass of water and urged me to drink.

"I don't know what it was . . ." I told them between sips, "if it was the candle light, the music, the deep breathing, or the ambience. But I feel as if I've just come out of sedation."

Paulette looked satisfied. "It was the Reiki."

That afternoon, as my fever spiked, I lay in bed, trying to recreate the sedated state that I had experienced on the Reiki table. Envisioning the shining, healing light as it wound its slow course through every corner of my body, I placed my own hands on the top of my head. I strained to remember the opening notes of the music which Paulette had played – the notes which were repeated again and again in the first movement of Paulette's Reiki CD – like a hypnotic incantation. Once they were recalled, I repeated them over and over in my mind. The telephone rang.

"Hi! How did it go?" Debbie wanted to know what the Reiki session had been like.

"It was remarkable. Like being sedated without drugs." I explained to her about envisioning a healing light.

"What are you doing now?" she asked.

"I'm lying here in bed trying to recreate it all, drawing in the light with every breath I take."

Memorial Sloan Kettering. They're all business and as efficient as a well-oiled machine. Efficient, but quite busy. Our appointment with Dr. Wong was for 8:30 a.m. We went up to the third floor which housed the Department of Gastro-Intestinal Cancers. It took at least three hours to get registered – to fill out address forms so that the films we brought could be returned to us by mail, waiting nervously in their spacious, nicely appointed reception area – until we were ushered into the clinic.

No one in this hospital will ever tell you outright that you'll do well. This was not Dr. Salwitz's office. Here, they were probably trained not to give "false hope." The atmosphere was very intimidating. One of Dr. Wong's fellows, a young Asian doctor, took down my history. She said that Dr. Wong was currently reading my radiology reports and looking at my films. Then she explained about the double, rectal-liver surgery which they do.

"It's a long surgery, and afterwards you're gonna feel like you were hit by a truck, but it's only one surgery, not two. That's a great advantage, because there's less risk for infection the fewer times you're cut open."

That made perfect sense. I silently wondered what it would feel like to be hit by a truck. Then I remembered what Dr. Salwitz had said.

"My oncologist in New Jersey said that this kind of double surgery isn't done because 'one place is clean and the other is dirty.'" I was wary of any procedures which might be unsafe.

She looked at me as if I had two heads.

"Well, we do this type of surgery all the time and have had great success with it. If you like, I can show you a study which we've done on it."

After this conversation, I was instructed to change into a robe in the adjacent bathroom and come out to sit on the examination table. Dr. Wong would be in shortly to perform a scope exam of my rectum and lower colon for which I had prepared at home by taking two enemas as instructed.

A technician came into the room and asked me to lie down on my side on the exam table. He inserted a tube into my rear and pumped a clear liquid into me, performing a "rectal flush" on my bowels. They felt like they would explode from the pressure. It was a preview of what was to come.

Dr. Wong entered, along with the fellow and a nurse. He was a quiet, tall gentleman, perhaps in his late fifties. We shook hands, and he explained about the exam he was about to perform on me. Lying on my side on the examination table, I assumed the fetal position. What followed can be likened to medical sodomy. I breathed slowly and deeply to get through the awful pressure which the scope exerted on my bowels. To distract myself, I watched the black and white screen which displayed an image of my innards in live time as the medical staff murmured among themselves.

"How extensive is it?"

"It looks like it's gone beyond the rectum."

"Is it in the vagina?"

They weren't talking about the scope but about the tumor. I lay still on the exam table, submitting to their probing, feeling my reflexes go on high alert as I caught snippets of their conversation. Closing my eyes tightly, I concentrated on my breathing.

Finally, they removed the scope, and I breathed out in relief. Dr. Wong gently wiped my bottom with a wet wipe, then told me to get dressed and to wait with Mike in his consultation room.

It felt as if we were waiting forever. We amused ourselves by looking out at the office workers in a neighboring glass-walled building, but our hearts thumped heavily, ticking off the minutes. Finally, Dr. Wong entered with his nurse. We stood up, full of worried anticipation. Dr. Wong was quiet and grave.

"The cancer has spread past the wall of the rectum into the pelvic cavity. I'm going to order a full body PET scan so we can get a better idea of how far it has spread."

I told him that Dr. Salwitz had already done so. He nodded.

"I want you to make an appointment as soon as possible to see Dr. Ilson, one of our oncologists. Dr. Ilson will set up a chemotherapy protocol. I think you should have chemo, followed perhaps by a course of radiation to try to shrink the rectal tumor, and then as far as surgery goes, we'll see. You may or may not need a permanent colostomy."

He spoke in the hushed tones of a funeral director. Mike and I stood there like dazed and cornered quarry.

Dr. Wong continued, "I want you to come back to see me in two months, and I'll examine you to see how you've responded to the chemo. We'll take another CAT scan then to assess your response. I also want you to make an appointment three months from now to see Dr. Fong, our liver surgeon."

It was a lot to digest, and my mind was swimming in an unfamiliar sea of medical uncertainty. To steady myself, I tried to focus on the particular and the practical.

"Can I have the PET scan done locally?"

He nodded yes, as the films and reports we had brought to him, taken at a local radiography clinic, had been reliable.

"What stage cancer do I have?" I was so thick. Everything had to be spelled out for me.

"Stage four."

Our mouths went dry.

During our car ride home, we tried to distract ourselves by listening to talk radio. Who should we hear but Dr. Stark! He was a call-in guest on *The Dennis and Judi Show.*

"Maybe you should call Dr. Stark when we get home," suggested Mike. "Just to get his perspective."

Stunned by the trauma of my first visit to Memorial Sloan Kettering, my voice was immobilized and I only nodded. When we got home, Mike, very tired from the whole ordeal and from the long drive, went straight upstairs to take a nap. But as for me, I was so devastated by Dr. Wong's grim assessment and by his quiet, grave manner in delivering it, that I just sat down at the kitchen table, buried my face in my hands, and wept.

"Ruth, you *will* get well." Dr. Stark was talking to me on the phone. I realized after all that I did need more moral support. Thank G-d he returned my call later that evening.

"Most of fighting cancer is mental. It's sixty percent mental. Your attitude plays a major role. Always remember that. You can overcome this, and you will. You've already started the ball rolling. You are going to get the best treatment, and you will get well."

My spirit soared skyward. The positive, encouraging words of a medical professional are a very powerful drug. Dr. Stark infused this drug into me, and at that moment I began to believe that I could survive.

Cancer can put you on an emotional rollercoaster, where you can be confident and hopeful one week, then sink down into despair when you receive a setback. From time to time during my coming treatment, I would call Dr. Stark, just so I could hear from him the words which filled me with hope and belief: Ruth, you will get well.

I was lying in bed, feverish, one afternoon shortly afterward, talking on the phone to Debbie. My two cats were on the bed, one at my feet and the other by my side. This was how we now spent our afternoons. Whether they were there to comfort me or to take advantage of the great heat which was radiating from me, I couldn't be sure.

"I don't want him to touch me." I was referring to Dr. Wong, whose quiet, somber manner had spooked me.

"I understand how upset you are," said Debbie. "But bedside manner is not what you should be looking for in a surgeon. You need someone with a high level of skill – someone with good hands. To hell with his personality! That's not what's important here."

I had to agree, but it was hard for me to get past my emotional reactions. Mike then burst into the room, waving a large envelope and giving me a big smile and the thumbs up sign.

"Hold on, Debbie, I have to look at some mail."

Mike had already opened it. It was from the National Board for Certification in Occupational Therapy. I examined the letter and the certificate.

"Congratulate me, Debbie. I am now an occupational therapist." I had achieved my goal – but not really, for while all my former classmates were now employed in the field, I had another, bigger challenge to overcome. A scene from a movie popped into my mind – the scene in *Von Ryan's Express*, where Frank Sinatra's character runs along the train tracks with his arm extended toward his fellow POW escapees, trying to reach the last car of the train which is pulling away from him.

Debbie was ecstatic for me, as was Mike. Later that day, in an email to my former fellow students, I told them of my good news – of finally becoming an OT – and of the bad news – being newly diagnosed with stage four colorectal cancer. Several of them would email me periodically, giving me much needed encouragement. Jen was always writing to find out how I was doing. Avigael sent me a new prayer book with my name engraved in Hebrew on the cover. I began to put this book to good use. Anna sent me a little gift – a small box, on the cover of which was printed "Believe." It was filled with inspirational quotes. This box became another weapon in my arsenal, and I would read through it as I lay in bed every morning, mulling over the messages contained within.

Events were now snowballing. Two days later I was in the nuclear medicine department of Robert Wood Johnson University Hospital. The liver MRI, ordered by Dr. Salwitz, definitely indicated a rather large tumor. Now he wanted me to have a liver biopsy to confirm whether this tumor was a metastasis stemming from the cancerous cells in the rectum. You must remain awake during such a biopsy, because you have to be able to hold your breath on command.

The surgical team was lively and bantered cheerfully with me. One nurse seemed to be assigned solely to be my coach. She held my hand as I was told by the surgeon to take a deep breath.

"Don't look."

I held my breath, tensed my jaw, and locked my gaze onto the nurse's. The surgeon, guided by an ultrasound-produced screen image, inserted a thin needle into my upper abdomen, into the lower right lobe of my liver, to deliver lidocaine to numb the area. The nurse's hands, clasping mine, were like an anchor mooring my attention away from this unpleasant business. After about ten minutes, the surgeon inserted another series of needles to extract liver tissue. These needles didn't hurt as much as the first one. Thankfully, it was all over in about another fifteen minutes.

"You guys were great," I announced, after it was all done. "But I hope we never meet like this again."

The following week, Mike and I were in the office of Dr. Z, the gastro-intestinal surgeon who had operated on Arlene, Debbie's neighbor.

"Because of his skill," Arlene had said, "he was able to avoid giving me a permanent colostomy."

After filling out the initial office forms and waiting a bit, I was brought into Dr. Z's examination room. I looked around for a camera-guided scope, but saw no such instrument. After disrobing from the waist down, as instructed by the nurse, I donned a paper robe. Dr. Z soon entered. He was a tall, balding, middle aged man with a goatee. He was accompanied by a female physician's assistant. After introducing himself and speaking briefly to me, he asked me to bend over and lean on the examination table for a digital rectal exam. It was uncomfortable, but nothing like what Dr. Wong had done.

Afterward, as we sat before him in his consultation room, Dr. Z began to read my radiography reports. All my films still sat untouched in a bag at my feet. Dr. Z hadn't even seen them yet. Mike and I looked at each other.

"Your tumor is six centimeters from the anal verge. Because it's so close to the opening, you will need a colostomy. I'm afraid it's unavoidable."

"A permanent one?"

"Yes. After about a two month recovery period, you should have your liver surgery."

Feeling shattered, I stumbled as I told Dr. Z about Dr. Wong's proposal that I first start with a course of chemo and then perhaps radiation. Dr. Z shook his head.

"The chemo will have no effect on the liver tumor. Since it's a vital organ, we have to get to the liver ASAP. But that means removing the rectal tumor first, for that is the primary tumor from which your secondary tumor has metastasized."

"Couldn't I have both surgeries at the same time?" I asked.

"You'd be under anesthesia for too long. It's too dangerous."

I absorbed everything he said. But mostly, I absorbed what he did not do. He did not give me a very thorough exam. He did not take the time to study my reports before examining me. He hadn't even looked at my films.

"Don't you want to see my films?" I asked.

He shook his head. "Not necessary."

Mike and I discussed our visit to Dr. Z during our car ride home. My case was more complicated than Arlene's. Perhaps Dr. Z had been able to avoid giving her a permanent colostomy, but he apparently lacked the skill to avoid it with me. At least Dr. Wong had not said that I would *definitely* need a permanent colostomy. Debbie was right. When you're unconscious on an operating table, the surgeon's skill level is of primary importance and his personality does not matter. The choice was now obvious.

The next day, I had a PET scan, a test in which radioactive sugar is injected into a vein. After sitting quietly for about forty minutes, you then lie still in a huge donut-shaped device, holding your breath when instructed by the technician over the loudspeaker. The test itself takes about fifteen minutes. Any malignant tumors will quickly take up the sugar, and the radioactivity will show up in the films.

On the way out of the testing room, I passed a glass wall, behind which were a few technicians looking at my PET scan slides on computer monitors. Inadvertently, I caught sight of several chilling computer images. A huge part of my liver was glowing pink, and there was a considerable pink mass in my rectum, out of which sprouted a large, tangled, pink web. Drawn to these ominous scans, I stopped to stare at them, as one would gape at an auto accident. There it was. Not only had everything been clearly spelled out for me, but I now had a candid snapshot of what was silently growing within. It doesn't get more explicit than that.

The Process

"I often wonder why G-d did this to me."

I was speaking to Paulette. We often were to have brief conversations during Reiki. It didn't seem to interfere with the process. And at this time, having had Reiki about twice already, I no longer felt anxiety during the daytime. But I sure did at night. As per Dr. Salwitz's report of my biopsy, the liver tumor, seven inches in length, had metastasized from the rectum and had been quietly growing in me all this time.

"Are you angry at G-d? That's a typical reaction." She had a lot of clients who had various illnesses and apparently spoke to them about how they were doing emotionally.

"No, I was never angry at him, even when I was first diagnosed. But I did feel abandoned by him."

"G-d never abandons us. Whatever he does to us is to teach us."

What, I silently wondered, could he could possibly want to teach me with such a harsh lesson?

"Perhaps," Paulette continued, "you should be thinking about what it is he wants you to learn."

Now that struck a chord. What did G-d want me to learn? I was to ask myself this question many times in the coming months.

The next day, Mike and I drove into Manhattan for our appointment at Memorial Sloan Kettering with Dr. Ilson, oncologist. But, first, as with Dr. Wong, we were interviewed by his fellow, a young Asian doctor.

"I would like to give you a digital rectal exam," he announced, after feeling my stomach and listening to my chest.

I sighed with resignation. "Whatever floats your boat." At least, when a doctor sticks his finger up your butt, it's brief.

Finally, Dr. Ilson entered. He seemed to be Dr. Wong's opposite. Dr. Wong had black hair. This guy's bald head was as shiny as a cue ball. Dr. Wong was slim. Dr. Ilson was pudgy. Dr. Wong was subdued. Dr. Ilson was upbeat. I liked him immediately. Dr. Ilson also gave me a physical exam, but thankfully, did not stick his finger up my butt. I told him about my daily fevers.

"That's from the liver tumor. It produces enzymes to which your body reacts by producing a fever."

Then we discussed chemo – how I would have a mediport implanted in my chest to facilitate chemotherapy, how I would be given Folfox with Oxalyplatin to kill the rectal tumor and Avastin to destroy the blood vessels which had grown around all of the tumors, thus choking their blood supply. His enthusiasm was palpable. Then, remembering what Dr. Z had told us, I asked if the liver tumor would be affected.

"About fifty percent of people have a positive response to Avastin," he said, meaning that this was the means by which the liver tumor would be attacked. "And somewhere down the line," he continued, "after your colorectal surgery, you ought to have a hysterectomy because cancer of this type tends to recur in the uterus."

If they had been able to put the mediport into me that night, I would have stayed until midnight to get it done. But these things require appointments. Could I have the chemo administered locally at Dr. Salwitz's office, I asked, with Dr. Ilson quarterbacking the protocol?

"Yes, but there's no guarantee that another physician will do exactly as we direct."

"Chemo, something else to look forward to." I was listening to Heidi, my cousin Jeff's wife, after I told her what was going on. She threw in this facetious comment because she knew a number of people who had been diagnosed with cancer and who had to undergo chemotherapy. It was not pleasant for them.

"I *do* look forward to it," I insisted. "Because I know it will help me." With every fiber of my being, I believed this. With every facet of my will, and with every ounce of faith which was within me, I told myself that I would be among the fortunate fifty percent.

Eight days later, Mike and I were in the New Brunswick office of Dr. Salwitz, and I was receiving my first cycle of chemotherapy, a process which took about three hours. Dr. Salwitz had expedited the implant of my mediport, which was done four days earlier at Robert Wood Johnson. Now I was all pumped up, like a boxer before a fight. As I sat in the recliner, Andrew, a nurse, explained to me what to expect.

"It's very important that you keep drinking when you get home. Even if you feel nauseous, remember to keep yourself hydrated. And if you do get nauseous, a lot of people find it helpful to take little bits of food because an empty stomach can make you feel worse. You'll probably feel fatigued and experience the greatest fatigue on the third day after the chemo. After that, you'll start to feel better."

Andrew also explained about the peripheral neuropathy – about how my fingers might become very sensitive to temperatures and how it might become difficult for me to do fine motor tasks such as buttoning. He explained about the possibility that I would get sores in my mouth. And he did not fail to mention that the effects of the chemo were cumulative – especially the fatigue – and would reach their peak at the end of the sixth cycle which I was scheduled to have about twelve weeks ahead.

To disinfect the skin, Andrew prepped my mediport with a yellow film, the smell of which, to this day, I still identify with extreme illness.

"Take a deep breath and hold it a moment."

He punctured my chest with the IV needle, pushed it down into the mediport and then covered the area with a clear tape.

Mike sat with me that first time.

"How are you doing?"

"I am so psyched up," I told him. It was true. The Reiki light – I envisioned it entering into my head, melding with the chemo and then transforming itself into medieval knights who joined me and, bit by steady bit, hacked away at the ugly gray blobs of tumors. Whenever Andrew came to change the IV bag, I asked him what he was giving me.

"This is the Avastin."

Ah! Now I could picture all of us slashing the blood vessels which fed the liver tumor, strangling the life out of it. In my mind's eye, I cut and slashed at them like a crazed killer.

Taking my IV pole with me, I got up to go to the bathroom. After using the toilet, I turned on the tap. Whoa. The cold water felt like ice. The chemotherapy was beginning to work its deadly magic.

They sent me home hooked up to a miniature, battery-operated chemo pump in a fanny pack, which I wore by day and placed next to me on the bed at night, its motor softly whirring and clicking as it delivered its noxious brew. My body gratefully sucked it up like mother's milk. Two days later, a visiting nurse came to unhook me, pulling the IV out of my port. In two weeks I would have my next cycle of chemo.

But chemotherapy is not quite as nurturing a substance as mother's milk. My fingers and palms became red and sensitive as if they had been burned. Often, I wore gloves in the house, because my hands would be icy cold. But I was fortunate, because unlike many people undergoing chemo, I didn't experience this neuropathy in my feet, and I was still able to stand and walk, albeit slowly and without energy.

Because of the chemo, cold drinks were off limits, for I would feel my throat begin to constrict and I was in danger of choking. Nausea became a new feature for about three days, which I dealt with by eating small bits of food at a time. During each week that the chemotherapy was administered, I would loose two pounds and gain back one on the following off week. Of course, there was the bone-weary fatigue which set in, reaching its peak on the third day after the treatment in the clinic. The fatigue never seemed to completely leave me, even during the off week. Entire afternoons were now routinely spent lying on the couch, for I was too exhausted to do anything except listen to music, read, or visualize my inner battle with the tumors. Fortunately for me, I was still able to do that. But it was hard to see the expressions on the faces of Mike, Zack, and Lia when they'd come home. My lack of energy distressed them.

And yes, it was emotionally painful for me to look in the mirror at the mediport site. It was flat and round, like a pacemaker sitting in a pocket of flesh above my breast, above which was an angry, red scar where the surgeon had sliced open my skin. Although the mediport was a clever device which was doing its part to save my life, it was also a symbol of illness which was now stitched into my body, changing me into a new, needy type of being – a patient.

As enfeebled as I was, I felt even more so when I was hooked up to the chemo fanny pack and had to sponge bathe instead of shower. As I washed, I would glance in the bathroom mirror at the outline of the mediport which sat just under the surface of my thin, upper right chest wall. The mediport was a kind of stamp which clearly labeled me, placing me among the sickly. And more than anything, I wanted to be well, to cross over that thin line which separated the ill from the healthy. I was like a hungry, homeless person standing outside a restaurant, faced pressed against the window, watching others enjoying their meal while I remained outside, famished and tantalized by the sight of food and comfort. How I longed to join them, those carefree, healthy people. Ages ago, I had been one of them.

"Oh, honey," said Paulette, when I told her how I hoped to be well within a year, "you don't realize how long this process can be. It'll take longer than that."

How I yearned to hear this one word from my medical doctors: remission!

But I was very ill and debilitated. The chemo seemed to have stuffed up my bowels. Either that or my rectal tumor had gotten to the point where it now formed a plug. In agony, my prayers now only consisted of tears of pain.

"Get over to the emergency room at Robert Wood Johnson ASAP," urged Janice, the nurse practitioner, over the phone. I called Mike, who left work early to take me to the hospital. Before he came home, I called my mother to tell her what was happening. I didn't want her to phone me later at home and find out I wasn't there. She started to cry. Now we had a change of roles. Don't cry, I told her, it wouldn't do any good. The doctors would take care of everything. I hoped.

An x-ray and a CAT scan of my lower bowels showed no blockages, but the doctor on duty did mention that I might soon need a stent placed in my rectum to allow the feces to pass out. At this point, I didn't even care. I would have let them do anything to alleviate the unbearable rectal pain.

After what felt like an eternity in the emergency room, the pain subsided a bit and we were sent home. As directed by the emergency room doctor, I then took a dosage of Dulcolax and Colace, two substances on which I would rely for the next few months, and I also ate several prunes. Now, it may seem bizarre to you that a person can be emotionally moved by a bowel movement, but the next morning, that's how I felt – overwhelmed with gratitude when my system finally cleaned itself out several times. Janice had told me that as the chemo began to take effect and kill off the rectal tumor, my bowel movements would begin to be more normal. I hoped that this was the beginning of that.

My friend Rhonda had brought over some food and a very good book, *Chicken Soup for the Surviving Soul*, after my first session of chemo. She had completely surprised me, for she worked in Valley Forge and had a long commute each day. Nevertheless, she had shown up that evening, concerned that I would be too weak to prepare dinner.

"Actually, Rhonda, the third day after chemo is when they say you feel the worst." But I couldn't believe that she had gone out of her way, after her long ride home, to get me the food and the book. It meant so much.

Well, I did feel quite crappy and, on the third day, even more so. But I spent a good deal of my time reading the great book that Rhonda got me. Mike went to Barnes and Noble and got me another good book – *Cancer, Shmancer* by Fran Dresher. I was to learn something from every book I read. In this one, I learned that people who are in good physical condition have a better chance of surviving long, dangerous surgeries and also recover quicker than people who are out of shape. I tucked this little fact into the back of my head. Another book, *Ninety Minutes in Heaven*, which I picked up in the drug store, was written by a pastor who had a death experience when he was the victim of a horrific car accident. He described his experience in heaven, which I found calming and comforting. Because I had a grave illness, I felt compelled to come to terms with death and find a way to embrace it, should an early death be my fate.

I started going to the library, borrowing books about cancer survivors and about people who had coped with and had overcome other serious illnesses and conditions. How did they do it, I wanted to know. What could they teach me? There was one book by Norman Cousins which had a big impact on me. In *Head First: The Biology of Hope*,

Cousins explores research into the effects of prayer, laughter therapy, relaxation therapy, positive thinking, and positive expectations on the outcome of illnesses. The main premise of this book is that one's attitude, thoughts, and belief – what goes on inside one's head – has a great impact on what happens in the body, for the mind directs the brain which produces hormones and neurotransmitters which control the body's functioning. There and then I decided that I would change my attitudes and thoughts in order to improve my own body's functioning. As Dr. Bernie Siegel urged in his books, I would look upon cancer not as an affliction, but as a challenge – a tremendous physical and psychological challenge. Along the way I was to learn that the psychological challenge of cancer is far greater than the physical.

Any little piece of bad news or even a negative image could send me into a mental funk. When I sat down to read in the newspaper that Dana Reeves had died of lung cancer, I cried uncontrollably because I knew what she had faced. In that regard, we were interchangeable. And when I watched the end of the movie, *Ghost*, where the main character walks into the heavenly light to be met by other spirits, I became filled with alarm. Was that the same light which I was envisioning during Reiki?

"No! It's not the same!" Paulette insisted. "What we evoke during Reiki is an empowering light energy. You know," she continued, "right now you're very vulnerable. It would be a good idea to be very careful about what you watch on TV and what you read. And if you should come into contact with any of that, don't focus on it. Just tell yourself, 'Delete!' – like pushing the delete button on the computer. Delete!"

Indeed, I was vulnerable and would have to be very careful about what I read, saw, heard, and thought.

I reasoned that I could not change my circumstances, but that I could change my attitude and my perception of my circumstances. Like an eager pupil, I did everything that Norman Cousins wrote of. I spent hours on the Internet, going through joke web sites to find things which would give me a good belly laugh. One evening, even though I was fatigued from the chemo, I stayed on a joke web site for forty minutes, laughing my butt off.

"You're going to laugh yourself into exhaustion!" commented Lia with amusement.

But afterward, I was able to stand and cook for two hours. Mike bought some funny videos for me to watch, but those did not make me laugh. Only the underlying pathos which surrounded each story and every character – that was what I now saw, and the tears would just flow out of me. Jokes were much lighter and, unlike movies, lacked the development of characters with whom to empathize. I began to memorize many jokes.

The following week, after my first chemo cycle, my pain was not so constant, and I was able to drive to Paulette while Mike was at work. It was a big step for me – to once again take a long car ride on my own. Paulette praised me for getting over the psychological barrier of venturing out like this, but really, driving so far on my own was more of a physical milestone, as it was my body which was behaving a little better.

I decided to spread the joy of jokes. Paulette said she could never remember any. So, as I lay on the table before she began the Reiki, I decided to tell her a very short one.

"A Black man was walking down the street and he sees a magic lamp. He bends down to pick it up. Out pops a genie.

"'I will grant you two wishes,' says the genie.

"The Black man thinks for a moment and says, 'I'm sick and tired of being Black. I want to be White.'

"'Okay,' says the genie. 'And what is your second wish?'

"'I always want to be surrounded by juicy pussy.'

"So, poof! The genie turns him into a tampon."

Paulette doubled over in laughter and sputtered, "You're crazy!"

"There," I said, tongue in cheek. "That one should be short enough for you to remember. You can tell it to your friends."

"I can't tell that to people!"

"Did you know," I said, switching gears a bit, "that laughter produces endorphins which boost your mood and that it also enhances the immune system?"

Not that Paulette needed any more endorphins floating around in *her* immune system. She reminded me of a statue of a laughing Buddha – her basic demeanor was joyfulness. In my life I have met a few very spiritual people, and I have found that those with whom you feel the closest connection to G-d are the joyful ones. Like Isaac in the *Bible*, who was only able to bless his sons after he had eaten a nice meal and felt happy, so too, all truly spiritual people are also happy. Paulette had that joyful, spiritual quality.

"I have no doubt," she smiled. "But it's time to get serious now."

She had to put herself into the right frame of mind to do the Reiki, and it was now my job to clear my mind of all thoughts and images, except for that of the healing light. It did require quite a bit of focus on my part. It was paying off, though, for not only had my anxiety cleared up during the day, but I also noticed that when I first awoke I was no longer anxious. It was only at night that my anxiety and fears crept up on me, keeping me from sleeping soundly.

I would have sworn that I never slept. But I know that in fact I did because I would sometimes wake up from vivid dreams. In one nightmare, one of my former professors sat across a wide table from me and a fellow student, criticizing our research papers. She told me that despite having earned my diploma and despite having passed the national exam, my paper was unacceptable and I would have to take two additional research classes in order to be an OT! I cried in rage and frustration, for it was so unfair to put a further barrier before me, and how I hated writing research papers! But she would not relent. Then I became depressed, but my professor still would not yield. Realizing that I could not change my circumstance, only my perception of it, I then accepted my situation and told myself that it was do-able and that two classes would not last forever. And then I awoke.

Alone, I drove to my second chemo cycle. Mike had wanted to come with me, but I didn't think it was necessary for him to take off from work for that. After all, the overpowering fatigue wouldn't begin to hit until at least the next day. That evening, I told him that I felt well enough to attend Purim services, with the portable chemo pump around my waist. Well, that was a mistake, for as we sat in the synagogue, I began to feel too weak to stand up. And in case you don't know, that's something that you have to do frequently in a synagogue. Then the terrible chills started.

"You look feverish," said Mike, looking concerned at my flushed face and glazed eyes.

After we returned home, I took my temperature. It was 94° F. I put my big, down jacket on over my nightgown and threw two blankets over myself in bed. It wasn't enough. Mike turned up the thermostat and lay down next to me, holding me in his warm arms. Slowly, the chills let up, and I slept.

But the fatigue factor was increasing. The next morning, after saying my morning prayers, eating my meager breakfast, and washing up, I went back into bed, bone weary as if I had the flu.

Arlene, Debbie's neighbor, had informed me about a telephone buddy system for people with colorectal cancer, which was started by a woman, Suzanne, in Texas. I had then called Suzanne. She told me that she had been living with stage four colorectal cancer for eight years and would match me up with a telephone buddy. My buddy, Sherry, now called me as I lay in bed, and we spoke about ourselves. Sherry had been living with stage four colorectal cancer for four years and had several small tumors in her liver, for which she was to undergo surgery in a few months.

That evening, I talked to Mike about these two women. To live with cancer for so long!

"Well," I said, "I suppose it's do-able. After all, people do live chronically with diseases like diabetes and asthma, and they still manage to function. And I suppose, if I had to, I could do it, too."

He nodded and held my hand tightly.

"But," I slowly continued, "even though it's do-able, I just don't want to be part of that club. I want to be free of it."

"Don't worry, Catsy." Catsy is his nickname for me. "I have a gut feeling you're going to beat this. And no matter what happens, I'll always be there for you."

That was true. Throughout everything so far, Mike had been the helmsman – inquiring about local oncologists, contacting Memorial Sloan Kettering, calling Paulette, and making trips to a local health food store for nutritional supplements, organic juices, and nuts which he urged me to eat. He was the man behind the scenes, propping me up, buying me books by cancer survivors – doing whatever it took to help me get well.

The possibility that cancer could become a chronic condition for me put a gloomy cast on the future. I knew that if Suzanne and Sherry could live with it for years, then I could too, somehow. But I longed to be completely well. Maintaining contact, I felt, with those who were chronically ill from cancer would emotionally divert me from my ultimate goal. Perhaps it was selfish of me, but out of self-preservation, I discontinued contact with these two women, although I kept them in my prayers. I only wanted to connect to and learn about individuals who had beaten cancer altogether. Those people were my role models.

"You could have a low white blood cell count from the chemo."

That was the assessment of the visiting nurse who came two days later to unplug the portable chemo pump from my mediport. "Whenever you have reactions like that, you must always call your doctor's office and let them know."

Well, it turned out that she was right, for the following week I was scheduled for lab work, which showed that my white blood cell count had plummeted. But that wasn't why I had gotten so chilled.

"You had an extreme reaction to the Avastin," said Dr. Salwitz after he had felt the lymph nodes around my throat. I was in one of the examination rooms at the East Brunswick clinic for my monthly exam.

"We're going to reduce it by a third for now on." He stepped back. "You look beautiful," he commented matter-of-factly.

I wondered if he told his male patients that they looked handsome.

I didn't want a doctor telling me that I looked beautiful. That was irrelevant. I wanted him to tell me that I looked *well*. But as certain as I was that I was not beautiful, I was equally certain that I did not look well, either. My hair, which had never been thick, was starting to become very thin from the chemo. After every shower, I would find dozens of hair strands clumped along the tub walls. So why the hell was Salwitz telling me that I looked beautiful? He wasn't my freakin' husband!

I was getting ready to leave the house for my third cycle of chemo, and was going to eat my lunch beforehand so that I wouldn't have to take any food with me for the three-hour session. But as I thought about the chemo and how I would feel afterward, a wave of nausea came over me, as if it were several hours post-chemo. It felt as if a stone were sitting in my stomach. Without eating, I drove off. After taking the precursory blood work at the lab, I waited to be seated in a lounge chair in the treatment room. A nurse came up to me with a sheet of paper.

"Your white blood cell count is still low, so Dr. Salwitz wants you to skip the chemo this week. Go home, rest, and make an appointment to come back next week."

I was so disappointed! All set to visualize destroying the tumor cells and the blood vessels which fed them, I wanted this process to keep moving forward. Now, I would have a delay. It was like denying my body its necessary ammunition. But I then made a mindful effort to repeat to myself the words of Rabbi Akiva: "Whatever G-d does is for my good." To quell my disappointment, I had to repeat this several times. When I got home, I realized that my nausea had vanished. I wolfed down my salad.

It was then that I fully realized that if negative expectations – i.e., the expectation that chemo would have bad side effects – could produce negative physical changes in the body such as nausea, then surely positive expectations could produce positive changes. I began to tell myself that I would feel fine after all the chemo cycles which were to come.

But I wasn't feeling fine just yet. Always I was so tired, and by evening I was exhausted. Beginning with early afternoon, I was still spending my time lying on the couch in the living room, either reading or listening to music or talk radio. My bowel movements were still very frequent and irregular. And then of course, there was the abdominal and rectal pain, especially in the evenings. Sometimes the rectal pain was so intense that all I could do was lie on my bed and writhe in agony. At those times I just wanted to die. Dr. Salwitz had prescribed a narcotic pain reliever, but I discontinued taking it because it made me constipated, and severe constipation is extremely painful in and of itself. So when I received information in the mail regarding my upcoming graduation ceremony (the second one, which I was eligible to attend), I decided not to go. I was still too weak to stand upright for long periods of time (which might be necessary during graduation), and the long, congested ride north on the Garden State Parkway to pick up my cap and gown would have been an agonizing challenge. So, for the second time, I did not attend graduation.

But the one week break in my chemo cycles became a turning point for me. Venturing out for a walk, I was actually able to go for twenty minutes before tiring. After one of those walks, as I lay on the couch, I noticed that a small wart which I had for years on the palm of my left hand was now gone. The chemo had killed it.

Since I wasn't working, I had a lot of time to read and think. I told myself that I would put myself completely in G-d's hands and be as trusting as a baby in its mother's arms. And, of course, I continued to go weekly to Reiki. During one of our sessions, Paulette suggested that I create a positive affirmation – a soothing, comforting, and uplifting saying to repeat and to have printed on paper in places where I would frequently see it. I thought about this, and told her about a poster which had been on the wall of the lady's room in a school where I used to work. Always, I had remembered that poster. It said, "Something wonderful is going to happen today. Expect good things, and they will happen."

"Perfect," said Paulette. "Write that down on several small sheets of paper and place them on your bathroom mirrors and on the dashboard of your car."

With Paulette's help I was able to create a detailed visualization to soothe my pain. My vision consisted of a long, soft ribbon of green moss which slowly wrapped itself in and around my bowels, all the while oozing a healing eucalyptus ointment.

"What do you think of that?" I asked Mike for his opinion of my anti-pain visualization.

"Very erotic," he responded.

When my pain was of a moderate level, I was able to control it with this imagery, but I found that when my pain was intense, I was unable to concentrate and visualize.

Gradually, as I attended the weekly Reiki sessions, the last vestiges of my anxiety vanished. And finally, I was able to sleep soundly. The Reiki had such a positive effect on me that I wanted to learn how to do it. Perhaps, when I would work as an OT, I could help my clients by doing Reiki to them. I asked Paulette if she would teach it to me.

"You're not ready yet," she answered flatly.

Now what the hell did she mean by that? Irked by this cryptic answer, I bit my tongue and accepted what she said. I would have to be patient.

Over the course of the next several weeks, an extraordinary thing began to occur: Although I resumed chemo, I began to feel well, and my energy level started to return. My fever subsided, and I started going out for daily walks – even when I was hooked up to my portable pump. After a few weeks, I was walking nearly as fast and as far as I used to. Instead of having to rest for entire afternoons, now I only needed to rest for an hour or two each day. And although my hair became thinner, I was far from being completely bald. Finally, whether it was from visualization or from the chemo, I was no longer in so much pain. To what do I attribute all this? Perhaps it was because the Avastin was reduced by one third. Perhaps it was due to the fact that I made an effort to go out and walk, and lots of people in the health professions will tell you that although it is counterintuitive, some exercise actually does make you feel better and can prevent fatigue. Perhaps it was attributed to visualization, positive thinking, and my Internet laughter "therapy." Paulette said it was because of everything, and the Reiki, too. I knew that, yes, all these things played a part, but ultimately what was happening was simply due to the will of G-d and to the prayers of the many people who were thinking of me.

Then, one night in early April, I woke up feeling very strange, as if a great force were taking over my body. It reminded me of how it felt to go into labor: You feel as if an outside power were directing your body with waves of energy. It was alarming. As I lay there, I quieted my mind and tried to figure out what was going on. An intense heat, starting in my head, spread over me, and I began to sweat profusely. And then I understood. I was having my first hot flash. I hadn't had my period since February. This was menopause. My nights of deep, sound sleep were to come to an end, for nighttime wakefulness and frequent hot flashes would soon become the norm.

"That's one of the side effects of chemo – menopause," Dr. Stark explained over the phone. I had called him just to hear his deep, reassuring voice reinforce within me the message that I would indeed get well.

"If you were younger, your periods would stop while you're on chemo and then probably resume. But at your age, the chemo just takes you straight through."

Menopause. I suppose that I could have sat down and mourned the loss of a part of myself. And under normal circumstances, I surely would have. But after feeling so ill during the previous three and a half months, I was now starting to feel so well that I would never even think to look back.

We returned to Dr. Wong on the first Monday in April. The somberness of our initial visit was still fresh in my mind, and I didn't sleep well the night before. My heart pounded against my rib cage as we sat in the waiting room, and I tried to calm myself by breathing deeply while slowly rubbing my temples. Finally, we were called into the clinic, and I was instructed to undress from the waist down, don a robe and make myself comfortable on the examination table.

How had I been feeling, asked the nurse as she entered the exam room. It was either a nurse or a fellow who preceded the entrance of the big gun doctors at Memorial Sloan Kettering.

Thank G-d, fine, I answered. Much better than before. Not so tired, and I was no longer running a fever.

The nurse went out to fetch Dr. Wong. He greeted me with his quirky, tight, little smile. After a brief handshake and the preliminary inquiry of how I was feeling, Dr. Wong explained that this time he would simply do a digital rectal exam. I sat on the examination table, pursing my lips as I stared down at his fingers. I sighed. They were long and moderately thick.

"If you were a woman," I noted wryly, "you'd have nice *thin* fingers." Then I lay down on my side and breathed deeply. This exam was thankfully brief.

When I sat up, Dr. Wong gave his verdict.

"Your tumor has shrunk somewhat. You'll continue with the chemo and make an appointment to see me again in three months."

A tremendous boulder had just been rolled off my shoulders. A positive response to the chemo! I then looked up at Dr. Wong, and there he was looking back down at me, smiling warmly. He said nothing further – as I've told you, the doctors at Memorial Sloan Kettering are very guarded in giving a prognosis. But the feeling which emanated from his eyes to mine could be summed up in one wonderful word: hope.

Now that I was feeling well enough, I made the long drive to finally pick up my diploma. My mother prodded me to take care of the paperwork for my OT license. "This way, when you're well, you'll be ready to go," she said. You can get "chemo brain" from chemotherapy and feel mentally sluggish. For a while now, I hadn't been able to focus my mind enough to even reconcile my checkbook. It was too detailed a task. But I now made an effort to download and complete the licensure paperwork, got myself fingerprinted, and sent out all the required documentation. A few weeks later, I received a postcard from the State Licensing Board, asking that I describe in writing my activities since December 2005. So I told them. In detail. They were probably sorry they ever asked.

Never had I been a gym rat, but I knew that I was very likely going to have some major surgery not too long from now. Remembering what I had read about how physical fitness affected one's chances of surviving surgery, I decided to go to the gym to get in shape for it. Mike wholeheartedly supported me (he had been going to the local gym for years), got me a ten day pass so that I could try it out, and went along to orient me to all the equipment that I would be using. We stepped onto side-by-side ellipticals, and Mike showed me how to program mine.

"Put it up to level ten. Go on; you can do it."

So I cranked the machine up to level ten. How the hell does he do it? I wondered. I was able to stay on for fourteen minutes before exhausting myself. Mike then showed me the various weight machines on the express line which worked most of the major muscle groups and the assisted pull-up/dip machine. After trying them out, I decided to put all of them into my new regimen. When the ten day pass expired, Mike got me an early Mother's Day present of a year's gym membership. It was the best gift I ever got, and I was to put it to good use.

When they sign you up in this club, you're brought into the office of the trainer manager, who asks you about your goals in the gym. When he asked me what mine were, I smiled to myself. My goals were not the typical ones which he must have heard dozens of times. I was not interested in taking two inches off my waist or losing five pounds or fitting into a size two. My goals were a little more basic.

"Well," I began, "I've been diagnosed with stage four colorectal cancer, and I have a tumor in my rectum and a huge tumor in my liver. I'm going to have surgery in the near future – a very long surgery, most likely. My goal is to survive the surgery and to make a good recovery from it."

He looked up at me from across his desk. There, that must have been something new for him! It obviously made an impression, for his young face went serious, and he said, "I'm going to set you up with Bob, one of our trainers. All new members are entitled to a free hour session with a trainer. Bob will introduce himself when he sees you in the gym and set up an appointment with you."

Later that week, I met Bob while I was struggling on the elliptical. He looked like a tall, lean Trotsky with a thinning, receding hairline. Bob was very good at small talk and important talk, too, and had a habit of emphasizing his point with large hand gestures. I found out that he was about eight years older than me, was a retired special education teacher, and that we had grown up around the corner from each other in Brooklyn. We even had some of the same elementary school teachers, and we reminisced about them.

"So what are your goals for the gym?" he asked finally, as I continued to plug away on the elliptical.

I told him.

Bob paused a moment. "Those goals are golden," he said, "and with hard work, you will definitely achieve them. But I also want you to think beyond that to the future. Start to envision what you would like to achieve *after* the surgery." He made a large, wheel-like gesture with his arm. "Start to think about that, because your life will go on after the surgery and you'll need to develop new goals, both in the gym and outside the gym."

I nodded. I couldn't imagine what new gym goals I could possibly come up with, but I did understand that I would need to go on with my life. But for now, I was preparing for an Olympic event – an eventual surgery, and possibly an extensive one – and I was driven as an athlete is driven, as focused as a student preparing for the boards. To help achieve my goals, I had started going to a Monday morning pilates class at the gym with my neighbor, Ann. She had explained to me how pilates strengthens the core muscles of the body. Surely I would need strong core muscles when I was recuperating from surgery. Unlike the aerobics classes which were given at the gym, there was no jumping around in pilates, and the pace was a bit slower. As I still had some pain in my abdomen from time to time, it would be easier for me to keep up in a pilates class. The instructor ran the class like boot camp, and many of the exercises looked easy but were in fact difficult. But I was familiar with physical discipline, for when I was younger I had been a member of a Shotokan Karate club for six years, and I knew how to push myself when someone cracked the whip.

"But to get back to your immediate goal, the surgery," continued Bob. "Cardio is going to be the key. Cardio work, above all, will get you through it. And the key to cardio is duration. You know how in real estate they say that the three most important things are 'location, location, location'?" He emphasized each "location" by pointing with a finger. "Well, in cardio, it's 'duration, duration, duration.' I'm not interested right now in what level you're working at on the elliptical." He glanced over at the control panel. His eyes widened. It was set to level ten, which I then explained was what Mike had said I could be doing. I had no intention of lowering it.

"Duration," continued Bob, "is what you need for cardio training and for the endorphins. And you, more than anyone else in this gym, need plenty of endorphins."

I knew exactly where he was coming from. Exercise causes the brain to release endorphins, the body's natural opiate. And exercise boosts the immune system by causing one's body to produce more Natural Killer Cells.

"Weight training, for you, will be like the icing on the cake. It's not crucial and not the focus of what you need to be doing. But if you want to do it, I've got no problem with that. But get your cardio in first. And anytime you want to talk to me, I'll be here."

And then we made an appointment for my one-hour free training session.

In a panic, I ran through the darkened hallways. A large, monstrous, brown bear was chasing me, trying to kill me. He had been harassing us and all the neighbors in the apartment house where we used to live in Brooklyn, pursuing us along a labyrinth of basement hallways. The lumbering bear would try to attack anyone he came across, and he liked to ride the elevator, rearing up on his hind legs when the door would open for passengers. The only way to stop him from menacing us, I knew, would be to kill him by shooting him squarely between the eyes. So, as the bear slept in his bed, I crept up to him and pressed the muzzle of my rifle against his forehead. Just as I pulled the trigger, my hands shook, throwing my aim off ever so slightly. Nevertheless, I killed the bear, to my great relief. Or so I thought, for the next morning it awoke, this time much smaller, lighter in color, quicker, and with several rows of small, razor-sharp teeth in its now long, opossum-like snout. I had created a vicious little monster who was out to rip me to pieces. I ran outside, the opossum-bear scrambling after me. The bear then caught sight of my mother, who was down the street, walking away from us, and I knew from the way he stopped that he was now going to pursue her, and she would be easy prey. With a flicker of inspiration, I banged the butt of my rifle on the ground to get his attention and then headed down another street, all the while looking behind to make sure the little bear was following. Yes, he was.

And then I woke up, fully aware of the meaning of this dream.

It was after my fifth cycle of chemo when I was scheduled to have my follow-up CAT scan to see how the tumors were responding. I went into the radiology lab fully expecting spectacular results. After all, I now felt about eighty percent normal, and I had been focusing very hard on visualizing the healing Reiki light, as well as going on a murderous mental rampage to destroy the tumors each time I went to Dr. Salwitz's clinic for chemo. And over a period of weeks, I had been steadily increasing my time on the elliptical by small increments. Now I was able to pedal it for half an hour before feeling that I could no longer continue. Moreover, whenever I was on the elliptical, I was plugged into the inspiring music of Andrea Bocelli and was simultaneously envisioning further destruction to the tumors. Entirely hopeful that the CAT scan would look beautiful, I felt in control.

A few days after my scan, Dr. Salwitz called, and he sounded very hyper and alarmed.

"The results of your CAT scan came back. The rectal tumor looks bigger and the liver tumor is the same size."

My nervous system went into overdrive; like a roller coaster cresting a hill, my spirits took a deep plunge. The words of Dr. C, the gastroenterologist, echoed in my mind: "It's a very aggressive form of cancer."

"But, I'm no longer in a lot of pain," I protested to Dr. Salwitz. How could G-d do this to me? How could he toy with me this way?

"That's probably because the inflammation around the tumors has subsided."

Instead of listening passively to Dr. Salwitz, my mind went into gear. I had another good, independent resource: Dr. Wong.

"I'm going to make an appointment to see Dr. Wong, and I'll bring him the films and the report."

Salwitz agreed that was a good idea.

Once again despondent, I sat with Mike that night.

"Don't worry, Catsy," he said softly. "I know you'll get through this."

But I never believed in keeping up charades. And I had a very strong hunch of what my chances were.

"I have a gut feeling," I answered, "that my chances of survival are fifty-fifty."

A movie scene kept playing in my mind: *A Christmas Carol*, and Tiny Tim's seat at the hearth was empty. So, too, would my place be empty after I was gone. Tearfully, I acknowledged that despite all my hopes and efforts, G-d had other plans for me. I tried to envision how Mike and the kids would get along after I was gone. If he ever should need good advice, I told Mike, Debbie had a patient ear and was very deliberate and logical in her thinking. He sadly nodded and held my hand tightly, unable to speak now. We both felt the dark clouds closing in. As for Zack, I continued to muse, he had a posse of friends and would hopefully go to Mike with any problems. But Lia was only fifteen years old and still needed a mother. The thought of not being able to be there for her was the saddest of all. I thought of each of my friends – of their personal qualities and of the proximity of their homes to ours – and tried to imagine how suitable each one would be as a surrogate mother. Then I called Debbie.

"Make me a promise," I said, after I told her about the CAT scan. "I don't think that I've ever asked you to do anything for me before, except to pray for me."

I could feel Debbie holding her breath at her end of the phone, waiting to hear what I would say.

"Promise me that if I should die, that from time to time you'll call Lia and ask how she's doing and listen to any issues she may have. My mother is old, and I don't think Lia's comfortable discussing 'girl' issues with Mike. She's really a good kid and has never been a problem, and you'd probably enjoy her. It would almost be like having a daughter." Debbie had two sons.

"Oh, Ruth, don't talk like this," she pleaded. "You'll get well. First see what Dr. Wong says."

"But just in case – promise me."

And she did.

Dr. Stark was always there to coach me forward, so I called to tell him the latest news.

"Yes, you're right," he acknowledged, "your chances *are* fifty-fifty. But which way the scale tips depends on your attitude. Remember, this game is sixty percent mental. You can overcome this disease. It's a big challenge. Ruth, you can do this."

Ever since I was first diagnosed, my good friend in Israel, Esty, had been carrying around a small note in her pocketbook and had been asking everyone she knew if they were going to Jerusalem and if they could take the note and stuff it into one of the cracks of the Western Wall. The crevices in the Wall were full of such small notes – each one petitioning G-d for a blessing or a cure.

"This is just a setback," she told me over the phone. "It's not the end. Try to see it as just a setback. And Ruth, I finally found someone who's going to Jerusalem."

This cheered me a bit, and I was grateful. But really, if G-d was determined to toy with me like a cat toying with a mouse, nothing would stop him. I then told Esty that I had joined the gym.

"You have the energy to go to the gym?" She was astonished.

"Thank G-d, I do. You see, having cancer is like being trapped in a maze. You're looking for any way out. I'm doing everything I can to get free of it."

"And, *im yirtzay HaShem* (G-d willing), you will. Instead of cancer killing you, you have decided that you're going to kill *it*."

That was my goal.

Mike and I were waiting for Dr. Wong in the examination room. He was reading the CAT scan report and studying the films. When I had spoken earlier on the phone with his nurse, she had told me that Dr. Wong had said there must be something wrong with the report, for according to his previous digital exam, the rectal tumor had indeed shrunk. Now he entered with his nurse, and it was the moment of truth. He gave me another digital rectal exam and then pronounced his judgment.

"The rectal tumor is unchanged in size since the last visit. The pelvic tumor is larger, but not significantly so. And the liver tumor looks the same – it's stable."

So was this good news or bad? It sounded neutral to me.

"What I suggest," he continued in his quiet voice, "is that you discontinue the chemo. How many cycles have you had?"

"Five."

He nodded. "I think at this point you've probably gotten the maximum benefit from the chemo and should discontinue it and begin radiation treatments to see if we can further shrink the rectal tumor so that your surgery will be less extensive."

With the mention of surgery, I thought about the colostomy – the possibility of which always hung over my head.

"Do you think I'll need a permanent colostomy?" I ventured. Back in February, Dr. Wong had said that I might need one.

Dr. Wong gave a slight smile, and answered in his quiet, guarded way, "I don't think so."

Although he didn't definitely state that I wouldn't need one, this shift in his opinion was huge, and yet another boulder had now been lifted from my shoulders.

Dr. Wong continued.

"I want you to have radiation for six weeks – that'll be five days a week for six weeks, coupled with oral chemo. I want you to make an appointment to see me a week before your radiation is done. Today we'll set a surgery date for four to six weeks after radiation ends to give you time to recover from it."

"When should I start the radiation?" I asked.

"As soon as possible."

He smiled his tight little smile, shook my hand, and exited with his nurse.

Radiation. Back in February, Dr. Wong wasn't sure if I would need it. And now I did. So, I would be totally encompassed by the cancer experience. But Mike had a good perspective on things.

"Look, Catsy, this isn't bad news. We're really back where we were back in February. Back then, Wong said you might need radiation. It's not as if something bad has happened. And he just said that he doesn't think you'll need a permanent colostomy."

"And," I added, now on a positive momentum, "The rectal tumor has shrunk since February. And I'm feeling much better."

"And you're able to go to the gym. So, things are much better than they were in February."

After I got dressed, we went to the front desk and booked the next appointment with Dr. Wong – and a surgery date, August 25.

"So how do you feel about starting radiation?" asked Paulette before we began our Reiki session.

"Well," I answered ambivalently, "I know it'll help me. But I also know that radiation makes you extremely tired. I'm not looking forward to *that*. And just when I'm starting to feel well again! Shit!"

She looked at me, amused. "You know," she advised, "it would help if you would envision it as a healing light. That'll help you keep a positive attitude toward it."

I nodded. I had read Dr. Bernie Siegel's book, *Love, Medicine and Miracles*, and among other things he wrote about the positive outcomes for people when they envisioned radiation as a healing force. I knew that I had to do that, too.

"And," I continued, "I have a date for my surgery. August 25."

"That's great!" Paulette looked thrilled, a feeling which I did not share. "And how do you feel about that?" she asked.

"Nervous."

"That's because now that you have a date down on paper, it's more real to you." That was quite true. She was very perceptive.

We began our hour of Reiki. Paulette placed her gentle hands, always newly washed before each Reiki session, on the crown of my head, and then over my forehead. They smelled fresh and soapy. I was continually amazed at the startling warmth which emanated from those hands. She said it was the Reiki energy. My own were always cold.

As I lay on the table I would usually have a series of hot flashes, and I would fling the blankets off of myself. Paulette had once coached me to visualize in detail a suitable scenario to counteract the heat.

"Ah!" I smiled, finally feeling some relief.

"What are you visualizing?" she asked.

"I'm lying in a bathtub full of ice cubes!"

"Isn't that a little extreme?" she chuckled.

"Not extreme enough! It feels wonderful."

Over the past few months, I found that the effect of Reiki was not merely deep relaxation. It had evolved into something which went well beyond that. I couldn't quite put my finger on what it was I was experiencing, but by now I felt totally calm all the time (except when I got what seemed like bad news), and well beyond calm when on the Reiki table. I looked forward to the Reiki as a junkie looks forward to his next fix. From the moment I got into my car to drive to Long Branch, a restful yet exciting feeling would wash over me. Upon entering the lobby of Paulette's building, I would begin to breathe in deeply the faint fragrance of that place. What was it? Just like the Reiki, I couldn't quite put my finger on it. Perhaps a subtle scent of lavender mixed with some cooking spices and a thin muskiness. The smell was more pronounced in Paulette's apartment, and I liked to inhale it and hold it in my lungs like the scent of a sweet smelling bouquet. This fragrance meant one thing for me – the profound calming effect of Reiki. It had become an integral part of my healing, and I now craved it. At home, I would often try to do Reiki to myself to try to get the same effects that I got with Paulette. It wasn't nearly the same. Let's face it, I told myself in the mirror. You are a drug addict.

Then one time after a Reiki session, I was feeling especially mellowed out, as if all was right with the world. This feeling lasted several hours. Early that evening, I had to go to the supermarket to pick up something. Not realizing that I was going a bit below the speed limit, I drove along easily in the right lane. A woman in a car tailgating me began to flash her lights and honk her horn. I had been oblivious to her. As she passed me when she exited the highway, she yelled out something nasty and gave me the finger. I felt my own anger begin to rise, but it quickly subsided. Normally, I would have bristled and would have yelled out a few choice words in retaliation. But this time, I didn't let myself get provoked. Merely feeling sorry for the woman, I wondered if she had been having a bad day. Now that was highly unusual for me. What was going on here?

And then, at the next Reiki session, I knew.

As Paulette put her hands over the "chakras" – the parts of one's body where it is believed G-d's energy enters – I had a very intense physical feeling of what was happening. I was being enveloped by G-d. It was a warm feeling of being surrounded and of being utterly and unconditionally loved and protected by a very great Presence. As her hands hovered above me, I told Paulette what I felt.

"Yes," she said with heartfelt concurrence. "Isn't G-d wonderful?"

She took no credit for what was happening. Reiki masters see themselves as channels for G-d's energy. Before doing Reiki on a client, they pray that they be worthy channels for that energy. That's what Paulette was doing before each session when she did that little ritual with her hands.

I was being embraced by G-d and filled with the infinite ocean of his love. And since I was just one small person and could only contain so much, some of that love, having to go somewhere, just had to spill out of me. That was why I was becoming more tolerant of others. After the Reiki, I told Paulette that if everybody could have Reiki done to them regularly, there would be no more wars. She agreed.

"Everyone should have Reiki done to them every day!" I reasoned. "Then the whole world would be totally mellowed out."

"We'd never get anything accomplished!" laughed Paulette. She paused and looked at me thoughtfully.

"And now," Paulette declared, with a look of complete certainty, "I think you're ready to learn Reiki."

Dr. Wong had wanted me to have the radiation done at Memorial Sloan Kettering, where he knew the radiologists, totally trusting their competency. But I didn't want to travel into Manhattan five days a week. So, I had Dr. Salwitz speak to Dr. Wong, and together they agreed that I could go to a local radiologist whom Dr. Salwitz considered to be highly competent.

And so I met with Dr. Soffin toward the end of May. He, like the other doctors on my widely scattered treatment team (except for the very subdued but highly skilled Dr. Wong), was very upbeat. He had a bearded, intelligent face – but it was a *warm*, intelligent face, and once again, I found myself immediately liking yet another doctor.

"How is your mother doing?" he asked.

"Thank G-d, she's status quo." Dr. Soffin had treated my mother the previous spring. She had developed a cancerous growth around her eye, and the radiation treatments she had received completely restored the tissue there. During that time, I had met briefly with Dr.

Soffin regarding my mother. As she was a very independent person, she had insisted on going to her radiation sessions on her own, via the county bus. Now I did likewise, traveling there by car.

Dr. Soffin then asked about my medical history and about what I had been doing to combat the cancer. As I had several times before, I started from the beginning, giving him a synopsis of how I was first diagnosed and of the treatment – both conventional and "alternative" – that I had experienced. He nodded in approval, even when I told him about prayer and Reiki.

Then he proceeded to tell me about what was to happen during the radiation treatments and what the possible side effects would be. Most likely I would experience pain in the pelvic area, diarrhea, and extreme fatigue. I might experience lymphedema – swelling in my legs. It could become permanent. He gave me a booklet which described in detail the radiation protocol and its side effects. And then, as do all treating doctors – whether it be those giving chemo, radiation, or performing surgery – he put before me a consent form which stated that I was aware of all the possible consequences and that I gave him permission to treat me.

I closed my eyes to all the bad possibilities and signed the paper.

We were being swept along in a series of doctor's appointments which seemed to have taken on a life of their own. The next day, Mike and I drove back up to Memorial Sloan Kettering for our appointment with Dr. Yuman Fong, liver surgeon. But first, before Dr. Fong made his entrance, I was interviewed and examined by his fellow, Dr. Cantor, a nice, good-looking, young doctor. Fortunately for me, Dr. Cantor had no interest in examining my butt. I told Dr. Cantor what I was doing at the gym (forty-five minutes now on the elliptical, plus pilates and weights), and I told him that I was no longer running a fever and that my appetite had returned. Dr. Cantor was impressed with all that. Also, I mentioned that I had recently stopped taking Dulcolax and Colace, and that my bowel movements were now nearly normal.

"This may indicate," he said, "that the liver tumor is either partly or completely dead and that the rectal tumor is partly dead."

Mike and I looked at each other in amazement, both of us suddenly infused with a new, hopeful energy.

Mike then asked, "Nutritionally, what should she be eating?"

"Plenty of fruits and vegetables. Lots of salad. Don't forget protein."

"What about vitamin supplements?" asked Mike.

"A daily vitamin is a good idea."

These doctors didn't seem to have any specifics on nutrition therapy. It was all very general, simplistic advice. Mike had been buying various nutritional supplements for me at a local health food store, but Dr. Cantor didn't have a clue about whether or not they were effective for anything.

Dr. Cantor also mentioned that I would need a radical hysterectomy in the near future, because stray cancer cells from the colorectal area like to migrate to the uterus and ovaries.

"Does it have to be a *radical* hysterectomy?" I asked. Dr. Ilson hadn't used the "r" word.

"Yes," he answered. "And anyway, your ovaries aren't producing much estrogen now anyhow."

"Maybe so," I countered, "but believe me, I need all that I can get!"

Then Dr. Fong entered. He looked like he wasn't quite forty. He was fairly short and a little stubby. His dark eyes, which shone from behind black-rimmed glasses, were very intense. Once again, as I had numerous times, I summarized my medical history.

"If this were twenty years ago," declared Dr. Fong when I was done, "we would send you home to die. But now we know the mechanism by which cancer cells from the rectum and colon metastasize to the liver."

He put the latest CAT scan films of my liver up on the wall in front of a lighted display screen.

"I'm one of the foremost liver surgeons in the world," Dr. Fong stated matter-of-factly. "I do at least five liver resections a week. People come here from all over the world to have me operate on them." He didn't sound boastful, but proud, like a schoolboy who takes pride in his academic accomplishments.

Dr. Fong looked at my films and continued, "I estimate that I'll have to remove about forty percent of your liver. I could take out up to ninety percent, as I sometimes have to do, and you'd still live. Your liver will be fully regenerated after three weeks. After another three weeks, it will be fully functional. You're going to feel extremely tired for about a month after your surgery."

"How long will the surgery take?" I asked.

"The liver resection should take me no more than an hour and a half. Dr. Wong's part of the surgery should take about four hours. After we open you up, if Dr. Wong sees that his part of the surgery will take four hours or less, then I will begin to operate. If he sees that it will take him much longer, then I may not be able to operate on you at that time."

We felt like we were being hurtled down the road of karma to the grand destination – major surgery.

Dr. Fong then began to quote for me statistics about the likelihood of survival and recurrence.

"Stop!" I adamantly interrupted. "I don't want to hear your statistics. I am not a statistic. I am an individual."

He was taken aback and began to stammer. I had apparently spoiled his prepared speech.

Dr. Fong tried again. "But, I just want to mention the statistical . . ."

"I am not a statistic!" I repeated hotly, tears starting to well in my eyes. I did not want to be a dead number but a living person. "I will *never* be a statistic."

Mike was appalled at my outburst. "Catsy, take it easy!"

Dr. Fong seemed to be at a loss, like an actor who, having been jeered at by a member of the audience, had lost his focus and forgotten his lines. After collecting himself, he once again began his statistics speech. This time, I didn't stop him. I figured he went through this lecture for all of his patients and didn't feel his visit with them was complete unless he had told them their chances of living more than fifteen years post-surgery. But I couldn't tell you what those statistics were because I never heard them. I simply tuned him out.

We shook hands with both doctors when the visit was over.

"So, we'll see you on August 25," Dr. Fong ended.

"Keep up your work at the gym," said Dr. Cantor. "Hang in there."

When I saw Dr. Salwitz later that week, I told him what Dr. Cantor had said about the tumors being mostly dead. Dr. Salwitz wasn't so optimistic.

"It's more likely that only part of the tumors are dead, as your CEA levels are still up."

Back in February, when I first came to him, my CEA level – the cancer enzyme marker in the blood – was 427. Normal is between 0 and 2.5. My level was now 265.

"But that's a good start," he concluded. Then he stepped back and casually remarked, as if to make it all better, "You're beautiful."

I was disappointed that he didn't have the same level of optimism as Dr. Cantor. And I certainly didn't need Dr. Salwitz to tell me that I was "beautiful." I needed him to tell me that I was "wonderful" and that I was doing great. Mike told me that I was doing great. Risa kept telling me that I was "un-freaking-believable." Paulette had been telling me that I was doing "fabulously." And Debbie would always tell me, "You're doing *so* well." At least Dr. Salwitz could have told me, as Dr. Cantor had, to keep up the good work. But he didn't even acknowledge my efforts in the gym. In my neediness, I craved constant validation and positive feedback. Just like good nutrition, I needed good words in order to thrive.

I decided not to focus on Dr. Salwitz's lack of excitement. Dr. Cantor's attitude was much more appealing. You may be wondering why, despite his lack of total optimism, I kept Dr. Salwitz on my treatment team. First off, we knew from various sources that he and his colleagues were top notch. But so was Memorial Sloan Kettering. It wasn't merely for the convenience of having a local oncologist that I stayed with him. I actually valued having differing medical opinions from separate sources, and I considered myself to be very fortunate that I could go back and forth between them and opt for the course of treatment which I felt was the most logical. When Dr. Wong's fellow had explained about the double rectal-liver surgery, we knew that was a state of the art procedure which wasn't available locally. Now, when opinions differed about the condition of the tumors, I could choose between my sources and go with my gut. And even though I realized that young doctors like Dr. Cantor tended to be more optimistic and more experienced ones were more conservative in their pronouncements, something in my gut told me to believe Dr. Cantor.

The following week, Mike and I took a ride to Boro Park, Brooklyn, to see Dr. Avraham Rosenthal, naturopathic nutritionist. Barbara had sent me a magazine article about him. He claimed to have experience treating people with various diseases. Although each day I ate a salad with at least ten different ingredients and took all the funky supplements which Mike bought for me, we felt that we needed some professional direction. Nutrition, we sensed, was the final piece in the puzzle to beating cancer.

Dr. Rosenthal was visiting temporarily from Jerusalem, and was using the basement in someone's home as his office. He was apparently religious – with a yarmulke and a long, gray beard. He wore a simple, rumpled white shirt and black pants. No suit, no lab coat. He was not out to impress.

As we sat across a desk from him, I once again reiterated my medical history. He took notes in Hebrew. After I told him what Dr. Cantor had said about the liver tumor possibly being eighty percent dead, Dr. Rosenthal smiled and said, "A miracle." He then looked at my irises through a magnifying glass.

"I don't see anything on the liver," he noted.

Well, that's not what my latest CAT scan showed.

Dr. Rosenthal prescribed a macrobiotic diet of only "living cells." Unlike a traditional macrobiotic diet, his consisted of fresh fruits and vegetables, a powdered protein mixture made out of almonds and other nuts and seeds, and a breakfast/dinner cereal made in a blender using whole, organic wheat, apples, dates, and some other fresh ingredients. No meat or fish or beans, nothing baked or cooked, and nothing hot, except for a cup of tea with a little milk in the morning. He also gave me a little squeeze bottle of a clear liquid and told me to dissolve two drops of it each day in a glass of water half an hour before eating breakfast. I asked him what it was. He shrugged and smiled, "Just take it."

Bob came over to me as I was chugging away on the elliptical, and I told him what Dr. Cantor had said about the tumors.

"Fantastic! Tell me, how many minutes of cardio are you doing now?"

"Forty-five."

"You need to be doing at least sixty to be in shape for the surgery," he said.

Sixty! It seemed like a big distance between forty-five and sixty, and it took a supreme effort for me to complete even forty-five minutes on the elliptical. Would I ever be able to do sixty, I wondered?

"That'll be my goal in the gym," I told him.

But whether or not I would ever reach that goal, or whether I would even be able to continue working out at all was questionable, for I was scheduled to begin radiation treatments in a week and a half.

Then I told Bob about our visit to Dr. Rosenthal. He shook his head. "That diet won't give you enough protein. I hope you're not planning on going on it."

I shrugged.

"Ruthie, you're very vulnerable right now. Really. You've got to be very careful about what advice you follow. I think you ought to go to an outside source – like your oncologist – and check out whether that diet will give you all of your essential nutrients."

Of course, Bob was right about checking things out and about my being vulnerable. Oh, yes, I was vulnerable in every way – physically, emotionally, intellectually – and I was ready to grasp onto anything with which I might pull myself out of the deep dark well which is cancer. And Mike, in his desire for me to get well, in his eager support of any and all paths which might lead us out of our maze, was vulnerable as well. Vulnerable. I had heard that term somewhere before. And if ever there were a single word which could convey the essence of what it is to be caught in a cancer web – that would be the one.

The Mysterious Will

I was on the Reiki table, in a state of bliss, enveloped in G-d's embrace, when I had a sudden insight. Looking up, I said to Paulette, "I know this may not be intentional on your part, but not only are you helping me to fight cancer, you're also helping to prepare me for death."

She stopped for a moment.

"Oh," she smiled. "I understand what you mean."

It was there on the Reiki table that I understood that the moment of death would feel very much as it does when one receives Reiki, only more intense. So, G-d enfolds you. I just know it will be so.

This new knowledge did not comfort me on June 2. On the morning of that day, Mike came upstairs with the newspaper. Having just awakened, I was still lying in bed.

"Read this," he said, solemnly. He had folded the paper to an article about a local small airplane crash.

As I started reading it, I came to the name of one of the four victims – Karen Nimrod. Who was that? I read further. She was the chairperson of the occupational therapy department at my school, where she went under her maiden name of Stern.

"Oh, my G-d." The words came out of me slowly like air from a deflating balloon.

"It just shows you," said Mike, "how fickle life is."

It was shocking, and I felt sickened from the news. She had been killed, along with her husband and another couple. I lay there, wondering why it was that she who had been so accomplished – a woman with a Ph.D., who had a family and a job where her influence touched many students – why she should be killed in one unexpected instance, whereas I, a very *un*accomplished person, was still alive with a seven-inch tumor on my liver. Was it life which was so fickle, or was it G-d? A phrase popped into my head: "senile delinquent." That's what one of Tennessee Williams' characters derisively called G-d in his play, *Night of the Iguana.*

That Sunday afternoon, we drove to the funeral. I felt as stricken as when I had gone to my father's funeral. There must have been over 700 people there – friends, relatives, colleagues from school, students, and occupational therapists from all over the state. And, of course, Karen's parents and two teenage sons were there. It was just too unbelievably sad.

"Why does G-d allow bad things to happen?" I asked Paulette before we began our Reiki session. I had told her about what happened to Karen Stern, and I was very upset.

"You mean, why did he let you get sick?"

"No. I can understand that. He's trying to teach me something. I mean, why does he let airplanes fall out of the sky so that people get killed? Is he trying to teach *them* something?"

She couldn't answer that, of course.

"Sometimes," I continued slowly, my throat constricted with emotion, "it just seems to me that G-d is crazy. I remember, back in school, we were in class discussing the tsunami of December 2004. And I commented, 'Here we are, in the middle of a sinking ship, and still the captain commands us to dance!' That's blasphemy, you know, in any religion."

"People are allowed to have doubting thoughts," she said.

"There's a difference between *having* thoughts and *voicing* those thoughts before a group."

"So you think G-d is now punishing you for that?"

"No. What he's doing to me – it's to show me." Perhaps to show me that he is a caring, merciful G-d, I thought. "But when he allows people to fall out of the air – now *that* I can't understand."

"Perhaps," said Paulette, "It's time for you to call Rabbi Labaton. Maybe he'll be able to answer your questions."

Rabbi Labaton was Paulette's Rabbi. He had gone through stage four colorectal cancer. I took down his number and said I would call.

That week, I began my radiation treatment. At a previous session, I had two tiny tattoos drawn by the nurse on the lower portion of each of my hips so that the technicians would know exactly where to aim their beam. I now lay prone on the hard treatment table under the radiation equipment, my face pressed against a sheet. The thin cotton robe into which I had changed for the procedure was now pulled up over my bottom. As instructed, I lay very still. With all my mental effort, I envisioned the radiation as a healing light which was entering my body. Nevertheless, I found it frightening, because – let's not kid ourselves – radiation is a powerful, destructive force. I focused as hard as I could to perceive it as a positive, healing energy, but was relieved when the treatment was over.

"So, where are you off to now?" asked the nurse, when I was dressed and ready to leave.

"I'm going to the gym," I answered. Probably I was the only patient there who would be doing that. Most of the folks in the waiting room looked so weak. For how long I would be able to keep up my routine, I couldn't say.

Rabbi Labaton sounded very upbeat over the phone. He told me about the four recurrences he had experienced, the treatments and surgeries he had undergone, his exercise regime, and his diet. But, my main concern was my question of how a good G-d can let bad things happen.

Rabbi Labaton sighed, "People have been asking that question for thousands of years. We really don't have an adequate answer for it. When Voltaire heard that there had been an earthquake in South America and hundreds of people had died, he became an atheist. But I don't want to live my life as an atheist. All I know is that I am happier believing in G-d, despite all the bad things that happen, than I would be not believing in him."

Despite all the bad things that happen in this world, I, too, feel the same way. I could not imagine what it would have been like to have gotten sick with cancer and not to have believed in a Higher

Power who had a reason for inflicting me with illness and who would guide me through it. This would be a learning opportunity, I believed, and much good would ultimately come out of it. Already, I knew that when all this was over, I would use my experience to help others get through their own illnesses. Always, I had assumed that when I became an OT, I would work with learning-disabled children in a school setting. But now that I was battling cancer, I wanted to help others who were going through similar ordeals. If I could help them, then perhaps this was the reason for my illness. But as for Karen Stern – I'm afraid I had no answers.

And so, I continued with the radiation therapy, five days a week for six weeks. Once each week I met with Dr. Soffin and had blood work done to monitor my CBC. Dr. Soffin seemed pleased that I was going to the gym during this whole time.

"You know," I mentioned to him, "once when I was on the elliptical, the batteries in my CD player died and I had to exercise without the music. I couldn't go as fast as I normally go when I've got music playing. It was torture!"

"That just demonstrates the power of the mind over matter," he said. "And, people who exercise during the treatment period also tend to have less of a negative response to it."

I had been driving myself to the clinic, which was located in a nearby hospital. On the way there and back, I had to pass the road which ran by the cemetery where Karen Stern lay buried. As I passed the intersection, I always found myself craning my neck in one direction, and I would start to ruminate about her untimely death and the senselessness of it. It was so easy to feel that if there were a G-d, he was indifferent to us, if not downright irresponsible – or even vindictive. Nevertheless, when I lay on the radiation table, receiving the invisible, deadly rays, I would turn to him and murmur, "Please G-d, be near!" Radiation was a fearsome force, and I needed to believe that a good, loving G-d was present, and would choose to protect me. Why me and not Karen Stern – now, that is a good question which I cannot answer.

"But, G-d is always near," soothed Paulette after I had told her about the radiation treatments.

"I know," I replied wistfully from the Reiki table, "but it doesn't always seem that way." At least, it didn't seem that way when something fearful, like radiation, was happening. It was only when I was on the Reiki table that I was able to feel surrounded by that Presence, and next to getting well, this was what I longed for most. Often I mused that, had I been born a Catholic, I would have become a nun.

At first, I felt no ill effects from the radiation. But, by the end of the first week, during the early afternoon, I experienced extreme pain in my pelvic area. If I caught it soon enough, I was able to take the edge off the pain with Ibuprofen; it was too intense for my visualization to be effective. I always made sure to get to the gym directly after radiation, before the pain would hit. And then, of course, came the diarrhea. Dr. Soffin suggested that I take Immodium to counteract that. Mistake! That stuff can constipate you, as I discovered, and believe me, I've been stuffed up enough to last a lifetime. So between the two extremes, I'll take diarrhea any day.

A week into the radiation, we attended the unveiling of my Uncle Eli's gravestone. He's buried next to my father in a cemetery out in Long Island. Most of my paternal cousins would be there, and we all planned to go out to eat at a local deli afterward. Mike and I arrived early with my mother and brother. As we waited for the others to arrive, I knelt down at my father's grave. The small shrubs which I had planted there at his own unveiling hadn't fared well, and the ground was now covered with dusty earth and small patches of crab grass. In a hushed voice, I spoke to my father, and told him what had been happening to me.

"Daddy," I said. "Gather the souls of all our dead relatives together." I then named them all. There were quite a few. "All of you – go before HaShem and ask him to let me live." My mother and two cousins each had a different type of cancer, and I also asked that they plead for their lives as well.

"And if you do this," I continued, "and I survive, I promise that I will return here and plant beautiful plants on your grave."

Standing up, I dusted myself off and looked around. The graves of my grandparents, twenty feet or so behind my father's, were overgrown with ivy, and I hadn't brought any gardening tools to trim it. So much for perpetual care in this cemetery. I'd get nice, short evergreen plants for my father's grave. If I lived.

In the mornings, I continued my routine of radiation followed by the gym and the weekly pilates class there. One day at pilates, I felt the pelvic pain begin just before we started the initial stretching. But oddly enough, the pain subsided and didn't return that day. And, then, another extraordinary thing occurred: I never experienced the dreaded fatigue. On the contrary. I became stronger; about halfway into radiation, I exceeded my cardio goal for surgery. One day, I managed to increase my time on the elliptical to fifty minutes at level ten, going at about 6.3 miles per hour, and then decided to just keep going. Now on a "runner's high," my fatigue faded into the background, and I reached the magic number, sixty. Bob gave me a big high-five to congratulate me, as I "cooled down" on the elliptical.

"We're going to turn you into a lean, mean, fighting machine. When you're on that operating table, you're gonna kick ass!"

I laughed lightheartedly. "I think that the surgeons are gonna be kicking *my* ass."

Bob then told me to add another ten percent to the sixty minutes, "just for good measure." So, five days a week, I did sixty-six minutes on the elliptical. Instead of listening to Andrea Bocelli on the CD Walkman, I listened to happy "party music." I had somehow come to associate the music on my Bocelli CD with Karen Stern, and I could no longer bear to listen to it. When the pilates class ended after five weeks, I continued doing the exercises on my own every other day, doing weight training on the off days. I wanted to be strong for the surgery. Now, why was I fortunate enough to have been able to do all this? There's only one explanation. You may scoff, but I can only attribute it to G-d's mysterious will.

That's not to say that I felt well all the time. There were days at the gym when I had to really push myself to complete my sixty-six minutes on the elliptical. There were times when I had pelvic pain, and some days I struggled. Depending on the song to which I was listening, I would envision my body destroying the cancer cells. The exercise was a type of battle in which I was now engaged.

Bob would often come over and talk. "If you need to slow down, do it. The radiation can take its toll on you. I'm not saying that you shouldn't obey your will – and it is considerable – but you have to listen to and respect your body, too."

When I felt weaker, I soon realized it was because my red blood cell count was down from the radiation, and red blood cells are what deliver oxygen to the body's cells. So, on those days, I would huff and puff and go a bit slower on the elliptical, so spent from the effort that I was unable to lift weights or do pilates afterward. And always, my routine at the gym would leave me drained for the remainder of the day, unable to do much of anything else. But I didn't care. I was a woman on a mission.

I was sitting on the examination table in one of the exam rooms. It was time for my monthly checkup with Dr. Salwitz, and I had come straight from the gym. Not having had the time to go home and shower, I was still drenched in sweat, and I suppose my face had a pink glow from over ninety minutes of exercise. Dr. Salwitz came in, and after asking how I was feeling and if I had any concerns, he began to examine me by palpating my neck and throat.

"You look beautiful," he commented nonchalantly.

Again with the beautiful! I had enough of that crap.

"Why can't you just tell me that I look *well*? Or *healthy*?" I blurted, trying to control my annoyance. My hair had begun to grow back. Friends and neighbors had been telling me lately that I looked good. Mike said so, too. Why couldn't Salwitz say it?

"Why do you have to tell me that I look beautiful?" I continued, my emotions beginning to seethe. "I don't want to hear that from you! It's so irrelevant."

This was the second time that I had taken a doctor by surprise. But Dr. Salwitz quickly recovered his composure.

"Well, 'beautiful' means 'well.' It's another way to say it."

He should have been a politician! But I wasn't swayed. He just didn't want to commit to using such words to a person who had cancer.

"If you mean 'well,' say 'well.' If you mean 'healthy,' say it! Don't say that I'm beautiful. I don't want to hear that. It's meaningless to me."

He continued to examine me as I silently fumed. Damn that man! Why couldn't he give me the positive reinforcement which I so badly needed? Well, if he wouldn't give it to me freely, then I would have to somehow wring it out of him. If it were the last thing I did, I would make him say that I looked well. I would continue going to the gym until I glowed – whether from just the thinnest veneer of good health or by the grace of G-d, from the real thing – and then he would *have* to say it. Damn him.

The Last Pieces

Nutrition – the last piece in my cancer-fighting puzzle. The one which, although I hadn't completely ignored, I hadn't pursued as thoroughly as I should have. Long ago I had stopped drinking soda, and I made sure that each day I ate a salad with at least ten different ingredients thrown in. I was careful to avoid processed food with the preservatives sodium benzoate or potassium benzoate, for it is theorized that these chemicals turn to benzene in one's body.

For a week or so, I followed Dr. Rosenthal's regimen. After running it by a dietician at the hospital where I was getting the radiation, I was informed that it was deficient in some essential amino acids. I discontinued it. Besides, Dr. Rosenthal's diet eschewed warm foods, and warm foods are comfort foods.

Mike had been buying all kinds of supplements for me and even bought me quarts of vile-tasting, freshly made organic vegetable juice which I drank unenthusiastically. He had never stopped nudging me to make an appointment with Dr. Simone, the cancer nutritionist whom Dr. Salwitz had recommended when I had asked him for a referral. So finally, the week after radiation ended, toward the end of July, we took a drive to Lawrenceville to see Dr. Simone. He was an oncologist whose sole focus was cancer nutrition. His office was small; unlike Dr. Salwitz's, the waiting room was not packed with people. There was a bulletin board on the wall with an old local newspaper clipping on it with a photo of a school boy. The boy said that his goal was to "invent a machine to cure cancer." That boy was young Dr. Simone. Now, nearly fifty years after the publication of that article, we were to meet him. We brought with us all the reports of every CAT scan and MRI that I had taken.

Dr. Simone wore a shirt and tie, slacks and sneakers, and had a very relaxed, informal manner. There were no other patients in his office at that time, and he gave us his undivided attention, noting my medical history, and that of my parents as well.

"You're Ashkenazic?"

I nodded. Colon cancer is relatively prevalent among Ashkenazic Jews.

He asked me about my diet and exercise. No, I had never been a big meat eater. Yes, I took one multivitamin a day.

"That's not enough. To fight cancer, your body needs more than the typical dosage of vitamins and minerals. It needs the right amount in the right proportions."

Dr. Simone then went on to explain that ever since World War II, because of pesticide usage, our fruits, grains, and vegetables no longer have the same nutritional content that they once did. Thus, we need to supplement our diet with vitamins and minerals. He espoused the following anti-cancer diet: no red meat at all – eat nothing that walks on four legs; low fat – fat absorbs environmental toxins; no soy – the isoflavinoids in soy mimic estrogen and they can accelerate the growth of certain tumors (I had been a big drinker of soy milk); no shell fish – not a problem, because I didn't eat it anyway; and take his patented vitamins, minerals, and supplements in the specific dosages which he recommended. Dr. Simone also said that it was necessary to exercise at least twenty minutes a day by walking (I was well beyond that), that spirituality was a very important element, and that it was essential that I get at least eight hours of sleep each night.

"I wish," I told him. "But I'm constantly being awakened by hot flashes."

"Yes, that's usually more of a problem for slim women. I would really like for you to get eight hours of sleep."

I would have liked it, too.

"What about supplements like green tea extract?" asked Mike.

"The problem with them," said Dr. Simone, "is that their production is not regulated by the FDA, and those products do not have set amounts of antioxidants in them. The antioxidant dosages can vary with each batch."

Then Dr. Simone changed the topic to one which he considered to be just as important as nutrition.

"And what are you doing for your soul?" he inquired.

Never had a medical doctor asked me that question. I always felt that they viewed the topic of one's soul as unscientific and therefore unworthy of discussion.

I told him that I prayed and recited psalms daily, and attended Reiki once a week. He nodded approvingly. We saw eye to eye. He asked that I keep him posted regarding my surgery, and to call him if we had any questions.

In a leap of faith, we purchased his supplements before we left. If I were to follow any individual's nutritional path, I felt it would have to be that of a medical doctor who knew that what occurs in the soul is interconnected with what occurs in the body, and who had dedicated his life to a nutritional machine to cure cancer.

The next day, I took a ride to Neptune to see Karla, a Reiki master teacher, to learn Reiki I. Paulette had explained that she was not qualified to teach it to me, but that Karla, who had been her teacher, was. So, after a referral from Paulette, I made an appointment with Karla to have an individual lesson in her home, after which I would be "certified" as a Reiki I practitioner. Not that I wanted to start up my own business doing that – I just wanted to be able to do Reiki to myself in the hospital after my surgery.

The weather was oppressively hot, but Karla's townhouse was nice and cool. She was perhaps a little younger than Paulette, with long, blonde hair, and she wore long, flowing, peasant-style clothes. Her home was filled with angel statuettes – this was apparently a very spiritual person. She had three or four cats which, like the deified cats of ancient Egypt, roamed the table tops and counters at will. In my house, such places were off limits to our two cats. Karla asked me to have a seat in the living room and to make myself at home as she puttered around in the kitchen getting food ready for her cats. Then she sat down by me, and we began to talk. Karla wanted to know about my illness, about everything that had lead up to it and what I had been doing since. As I had many times before, I retold my story.

"I noticed that when you speak about the tumors, you never refer to them as 'my tumors' as many people would," she commented. "It's a healthy thing that you do not look upon them as part of who you are."

"I never did," I replied. "I've always viewed them as foreign invaders whom I've had to kill."

Then we started to talk about Reiki. It turned out that I already knew quite a lot about it and its history, as I had read a library book on the subject. Karla then told me the story of a man who had become a client of hers. He was an atheist and had developed lung cancer. He was given a terminal diagnosis and was very much afraid of dying. His wife brought him to Karla for Reiki, and although the man was skeptical, he allowed Karla to perform Reiki on him. Karla said that during the session he began to cry; he told her that he felt a light and a presence all around him. After that, he became calmed and was no longer afraid of death. I understood exactly what he felt, I said, because, although I believed in G-d, that's just what Reiki had done for me. At least for me, I wasn't afraid of death when I was on the Reiki table!

"That man eventually died," said Karla. "Experiencing the light enabled him to realize that there is a Higher Power, and it allowed him to calmly accept death. But it's different for you. You are going to live. For you, the light is empowerment."

Totally focused, I listened deeply to her, making my mind and body believe what she said.

"And everything that G-d does to you is for a reason. You will come out of this experience stronger and wiser than you were. And perhaps, when you do have your surgery, it will not be so extensive."

"I don't think so," I answered. "I have a feeling that it's going to be *very* extensive."

"And why is that?"

"Because," I said slowly, "I believe that G-d wants me to know what it is that people go through. This way, I'll be a better occupational therapist."

I had come to this conclusion after much reflection. This must be the lesson which G-d wanted me to learn. Of course, I still yearned to be cured, but along the way, it was my task to learn and absorb, through direct experience, from soup to nuts, what it meant to be a patient – to know, feel, and understand all the fears, fatigue, hopes, and pain which severe illness brings. Karla just looked at me thoughtfully and did not try to refute what I said.

She then showed me a very unusual little book, *The Hidden Messages in Water*. It consisted mostly of photographs of the beautiful crystal shapes which water droplets assume when they are exposed to positive words and thoughts. Since our bodies are approximately eighty percent water, you can just imagine the significance of this. Positive words and thoughts can actually influence body structure. The most beautiful photos of water crystals were those where the water had been exposed to the words "love" and "gratitude."

"Now try to think," said Karla, "of a time when you felt especially grateful. Close your eyes and try to recapture that feeling."

That was easy. What came to mind was the day after I returned from the emergency room at Robert Wood Johnson and finally cleared out my bowels. Never had I been so grateful.

"Got it," I told her.

"Good. That is the feeling which I want you to focus on and cultivate. I want you to start every morning with that feeling. And when you do Reiki to yourself, I want you to concentrate on this feeling of gratitude to G-d."

Karla then performed Reiki on me as I sat in a chair. Afterward, she enacted an odd little ceremony wherein she bent her head close to my "heart space" chakra and "blew" the powers of a Reiki I practitioner into me. So that was it? Throughout the entire weird rite, I suppressed my natural skepticism and kept an open mind. After all, if this were to give me the power to perform Reiki on myself, who was I to argue? Karla even printed out a certificate stating that I was now certified in Reiki I. But there was one last thing that she did which helped me tremendously. Karla gave me some advice – a lesson in positive thinking.

"Instead of telling yourself 'I *will* get well,' tell yourself 'I am *getting* well.'"

And then she had me visualize about myself.

"I want you to close your eyes," she said, "and see yourself as you want to be, down to the last detail. See yourself as you want to be after you are fully recovered from your surgery."

As I sat on the couch, I closed my eyes and formed a detailed picture of myself in my mind's eye. Dressed in nice street clothes, I was strong, healthy, and full of energy, and I was working as an occupational therapist somewhere near my home. I had come through my experience stronger in every way. This image was so complete that it was like looking at a photograph of myself – of how I was going to be in a not-too-distant time.

"Now tell yourself, 'It's already done!'"

I did as Karla instructed, pronouncing those words with fervor, and in so doing, I knew at that moment that somehow, submerged somewhere inside me, there really was that healthy, vital person straining to be released.

August had arrived. Radiation had ended in mid-July, and now I was in the middle of an interval wherein my body was recovering from all the treatment which I had undergone so that I would be ready for the surgery which loomed ahead. The thought of lying on an operating table was unnerving.

"We'll schedule a pre-surgery session for you," said Paulette. "You'll be all right."

Even though I was now "certified" to do Reiki, and performed it on myself every evening as I listened to a CD of Reiki music which I had bought, my "powers" were nowhere near those of Paulette, and I continued to see her weekly for my spiritual "fix." It occurred to me that Reiki, meditation, and prayer were all related, in that they were ways for us to communicate with and feel the presence of G-d. And this I needed above all.

Before I was hospitalized, I decided to take care of a few things. To make sure my teeth were in good condition, I had made an appointment to see Dr. Rajam, my dentist, for my six-month checkup. After all, I certainly didn't need any additional problems while I was in the hospital.

He came into the exam room and greeted me as I sat back in the dental chair. Dr. Rajam was short and a little pudgy, with a dark, handsome Hindu face.

"So, how have you been? In good health?"

I told him my story. He listened with his mouth opened, astonished.

"But you look well! What have you been doing?"

Reiki, prayer, exercise, laughter therapy, positive thinking, Dr. Simone's nutritional regimen – I told him everything. He was listening intently, I could tell, because he didn't take his eyes off my face as I spoke. Rather, his eyes were locked onto mine.

"What you need to do now," he said, when I had finished, "is make your next appointment for six months from now. You will come through the surgery. It's important that you book your next appointment."

Yes, making a future appointment was a way to tell myself that I was going to survive.

After Dr. Rajam finished examining and cleaning my teeth, he gave me a sample of a high fluoride toothpaste to use at night in case I should experience dry mouth from any follow-up chemo.

"And don't forget to make that appointment at the desk before you leave! I will see you back in six months! Good luck."

Back in the gym, I chugged away on the elliptical, all the while envisioning my white blood cells attacking the tumors. Bob came over to me. "When is the last day that you plan on working out?"

"You mean, before the surgery?" I asked.

He nodded.

"The day before the surgery, of course!" I answered.

Bob shook his head. "That's what I thought you'd answer. And that's not what I want you to do. You'll actually be stronger if you stop working out a week to ten days before the surgery. Then you'll be at your peak physically."

As I listened to him, I continued to pedal the foot plates.

"Really, it's a fact. This was discovered accidentally when a marathon runner had to stop training because he caught the flu. He had to rest for ten days. After that, his performance time was even better than it had been previously when he had worked out up to the day of the race. Now all marathon runners follow suit. So, a week to ten days before the surgery, I want you to pull back. Stop going to the gym. No exercise for you."

His request left me feeling disappointed. After all, my preparation for the surgery had taken on a life of its own. I was driven, and like a wild animal, I didn't want to be reigned in.

"Can't I even do any pilates?" I asked hopefully.

"No! No pilates, no weights. If you want, you can walk – but I know *you*! You'll want to speed walk! Make sure you take nice, *leisurely* walks. Either that or you can just do nothing and sit on your porch in your rocking chair, and you'd still be at your peak. But no stressful exercise."

As I absorbed what Bob said, I continued to plug away on the elliptical. It was hard for me to accept, because I can become compulsive.

"Now, I'll be going away on vacation next week, and I won't be here to remind you. So promise me that you'll pull back."

Sighing, I decided that I would take his advice – I'd stop my routine seven days before the surgery, not ten.

"I promise," I said reluctantly.

Bob nodded. "I know you'll be just great and will breeze through the surgery."

"Thank you, Bob, for everything."

"My pleasure, Ruthie. And I'll see you sometime after your recovery, when you're able to get back to the gym."

After doing my weight training, I left for home. As usual, my tee shirt was drenched in sweat, front and back, evidence of the effort I had put in. There was still some time for me to go home to shower before my appointment with Dr. Salwitz – the last one scheduled with him before the surgery. As I headed for the door, I waved goodbye to Bob.

"Remember," he called to me, "pull back!"

I sat on the exam table, waiting for Dr. Salwitz. The wait was never too long. He strode in and began with the usual opening pleasantries.

"How do you feel?" he asked.

"I feel fine." It was true.

"Any pain?"

"Just an ever-so-slight pain where my liver is. Nothing like what it used to be."

He palpated my throat and then my abdomen as I lay on the table. I sat up and he stepped back, taking a long look at me.

"You look good!"

Yes! He had said it at last! Exultation began streaming through me like sunlight because of those three words which I now heard from him. Yes! I had thrown my all into preparing myself for the surgery. His words were the final vindication of everything I had done. What's more, I was once again getting completely positive reinforcement from a medical doctor, and that, let me tell you, is very strong reinforcement, indeed.

He felt my shoulders and arms. I didn't look like your typical cancer patient.

"Strong," he commented.

Damn right, I thought. Strong enough to knock your block off if you dare call me beautiful!

Then I told him what I had been doing in the gym to prepare for the surgery. Now he listened! He whistled.

"You should be the poster child for all cancer patients! If anyone can get through this surgery, you can, Ruth."

I hopped off the table, and he shook my hand.

"Best of luck to you. Make an appointment to see me two months after your surgery, when you're fully recovered."

In my readings in the genre of cancer survivors, there was a common element which ran through many of the stories: While undergoing treatment, these people prepared things for their future. They bought outfits for their children's weddings, or they made plans to go on a cruise. They actually made plans or acquired things which they were going to use for very specific events – and in so doing, by giving themselves physical evidence that they were going to live, they had a hand in laying the groundwork for a future in which they would be participants. And where the mind goes, the body often follows. For a long while I hadn't bought myself anything new. Inside me there had remained a small vestige of doubt, and I hadn't completely believed that I would live to wear any new clothes. So, what was the point in buying? But as I began to feel better physically, I started to think more about the future.

At a shoe sale, I went and bought myself an extra pair of sneakers, telling myself that I would surely wear out the ones I had now and would soon need another pair – and I would wear those out as well. And now, with surgery looming ahead, I wanted to ensure that I would have specific things to look forward to afterward. So, Mike and I went to Sims, where I purchased a lovely white suit for Yom Kippur and a navy pin-striped business suit for interviews – for after I was fully recovered from the surgery, I would look for a job, and I needed the tools to do that. I was laying the groundwork for the future. I came out of the fitting room to get Mike's opinion of the interview suit.

"How do I look?"

He looked me over and up and down. Except for the pants and sleeves being a bit long, it fit perfectly, as if it had been stitched together just for me.

"You look all business."

Sold. I'd have the alterations done before the surgery.

We also purchased tickets to a Broadway show. Mike would rather stay home and watch football, but I love Broadway. Nevertheless, he insisted that we buy seats in advance to a show – to give me something to look forward to. We got tickets for November.

After I stopped going to the gym, Mike and I went to Holmdel Park and hiked along the trails. Restraining myself from bounding along, I tried to walk leisurely as I navigated through the criss-crossing, tree-lined paths, using a map to find our way. I love to read maps, but I often make a lot of wrong turns in the woods. Fortunately, I have a pretty good sense of direction and a good memory for landmarks, and eventually find my way.

Before the surgery, I had to go to Memorial Sloan Kettering for a final CAT scan, to Dr. Wong and Dr. Fong to sign consent forms for the surgery, and for pre-op testing, which consisted of blood work and an EKG. In the clinic, Dr. Wong came in with one of his nurses. There would be no exam this time, just an explanation of how to prep for the surgery and the signing of the consent form. I read through the form. It gave Dr. Wong permission to perform an anterior rectal resection, a possible ileostomy, a possible total abdominal hysterectomy, a possible double oophorectomy, a possible pelvic node dissection, and a possible partial vaginectomy. During the course of the surgery, Dr. Wong would decide if each procedure was necessary. Oh G-d, I said to myself, please don't let all this happen to me. I felt like a turkey waiting to be carved up.

The ileostomy, if necessary, would be a temporary one, and I would be taught to change the bag in which my feces would collect. As I lay on the examination table, Dr. Wong's nurse marked a spot on my lower abdomen for the ileostomy incision.

Could I have Reiki done to me during the surgery, I asked Dr. Wong? Paulette had suggested it; she had performed Reiki in operating rooms before. Unfortunately, Dr. Wong hadn't the slightest idea of what Reiki was, but he did agree that I could listen to my CD. On some level, I had read, even when you are unconscious, your sense of hearing is not entirely absent. The Reiki music would help to keep me inwardly calm.

Next it was on to Dr. Fong, to sign his consent form. But first, a nurse came into the exam room to explain how I would be put asleep with anesthesia, with a breathing tube inserted down my trachea after I was put under, and a Foley catheter inserted as well. I nodded in resignation. All this was unavoidable with a long surgery.

We expected Dr. Fong to come in, but instead one of his fellows, Dr. Rebecca White, entered – a young, intelligent-looking woman, who explained that Dr. Fong was stuck in London following the terrorist subway bombings.

"He just better be back in New York on August 25," I said.

"I'm sure that he will be."

Then she presented the consent form, which had no other possible surgeries listed other than the liver resection, which I was to give Dr. Fong permission to perform. Perhaps, I thought, there was another Dr. Fong in this hospital, and this other guy would perform the surgery should my Dr. Fong be delayed in London. Taking the pen which Dr. White gave me, I added a caret, above which I wrote the name "Yuman."

"Dr. *Yuman* Fong will perform the surgery," I proclaimed. "Not Dr. Joe Fong. Not Dr. Moe Fong, but Dr. Yuman Fong." I wasn't taking any chances.

"We only have one Dr. Fong here," said Dr. White patiently. And then she suggested that we go down the hall to check out the films of my latest CAT scan. Mike and I bounded down the hall after her into a small office. We stood next to Dr. White as she brought the latest black and white views of my liver into focus on a computer screen.

"Do you see the difference in shading in the liver?" she asked. "Most of the right lobe is a dark shade of gray. This tells me that at least eighty percent of your liver tumor is dead." Dr. White looked up from the screen, her eyes gleaming from behind her glasses. Here was another ally for me, this young, enthusiastic doctor. Mike and I shot each other a brief, but meaningful look, for we were now excited with yet more hope. Nothing else mattered at the moment.

But, when I went later that day for the EKG, an abnormality turned up in one of the waves. This, as was explained to me, could be due to the chemo. But doctors like to cover themselves, so Dr. Wong had me schedule an echo-cardiogram at the hospital in addition to an examination by one of the hospital's cardiologists. I was mad because I just knew that there was nothing wrong with my heart. For G-d's sake, in nearly three months, I had traveled the equivalent of hundreds of miles on the elliptical!

The echo-cardiogram showed that I had a slight heart murmur, which I'd known about for years. As for the visit with Dr. Baum, the cardiologist, it was pathetic. He looked so worn out and overweight that my annoyance at having to come into the city for yet another exam melted, and I actually felt sorry for him. I didn't have the heart to even jokingly challenge him to a race around the block, because I didn't think he'd survive it. He took my blood pressure and listened to my heart, wheezing softly as he pressed his stethoscope to my chest. Then he cleared me for surgery.

That Sunday was my birthday. Coincidentally, my cousins Heidi and Jeff had planned a barbeque for our cousins in their backyard in the afternoon. It was like another mini-reunion, and they all wished me well on my upcoming surgery, which was now only days away. My cousin Selma had brought a chocolate birthday cake which had "Happy Birthday, Ruthie" written on top in white icing. I was touched. It had been a very long time since I had a cake with my name on it.

The afternoon slowly ebbed into beautiful evening, and we reluctantly said goodbye to our cousins. A week from now, I thought, I will have had the surgery and will be lying in a hospital bed. G-d.

In the Hands of G-d

Everything was in place. I had the antibiotic I was to take and the two little bottles of a substance which would clean out my bowels. The house was spotless and all excess laundry done. The last thing left, before I began the bowel prep, was to go to my final Reiki appointment before the surgery. It would be a two-hour special session which would hopefully calm me. Right then, I was anything but. Mike and I drove to Long Branch; he took a walk along the beach while I went up to Paulette.

We sat on the large sectional in her living room, and Paulette asked me to express my concerns about the upcoming surgery as she took notes on a pad of paper.

With the surgery only two days away, I was riddled with anxiety. Taking a deep breath, I thought aloud about what exactly it was that was making me nervous.

"Well," I began, "I suppose the most frightening thing to me is to be put asleep. I'm afraid that I won't wake up. And while I'm asleep, I won't have any control over what they do to me. I'll be completely at their mercy, and they could possibly make mistakes and do something which could kill me."

Paulette looked up momentarily from her pad with a poker face. She obviously wanted me to continue speaking, and she didn't want to appear judgmental. Paulette then continued to write.

"I'm really not afraid of what will come after the surgery – the pain of recovery. I know that I can get through that, somehow. I'm just concerned that I won't get to that point because I'll die on the operating table. Being put under anesthesia is very frightening to me – it's like being in a state of nonexistence. Like being in a state that is so close to death that it can actually *become* death if the surgeons should make one mistake."

Paulette nodded and continued writing. Then I thought of my mother. Earlier that day I had seen her in the supermarket. She had cried then, asking me why I had to have the surgery when I was feeling well.

"And my mother," I continued. "She's usually so logical. But today I had to explain to her, as one explains to a child, that I couldn't let the tumors remain inside me. They have to be taken out. It's as if our roles were reversed, and now *I'm* the logical thinking one."

When I was done, Paulette put down her notepad and asked that I go into the other room where the Reiki table now was, lie down on it, and either read or do Reiki to myself as she prepared herself for the session. Too tense to read, I decided to lie down on the Reiki table, breathe slowly and deeply, and perform my paltry Reiki on myself. I didn't have my cassette walkman and my copy of the Reiki CD with me, but you don't really need such music to do Reiki. A good Reiki session depends more on deep, slow breathing and on your ability to clear your mind of extraneous thoughts. By doing this, you become calm and aware of G-d's presence.

Right then, on the Reiki table, I was anything but calm. This must be what new soldiers feel like on the cusp of battle, I thought to myself. Only, I reasoned, soldiers must battle an enemy, whereas I would have two teams of doctors surrounding me, helping me, working for me. . . .

As my heart thumped against my ribcage, I put my palms along the sides of my face. Paulette had sometimes done this to me during Reiki.

Paulette came into the room and stood next to the table, looking down at me. "Are you Reikiing your ears?" she asked curiously.

Too nervous now to speak, I managed a curt reply. "No, my face."

She looked down at me thoughtfully. "Does that comfort you?"

How perceptive she was! Slowly, I nodded, keeping my hands locked around my face.

Paulette then gently grasped my wrists and lifted up my hands. She noticed the three thin karma bracelets I was wearing; Debbie had given them to me the other day, and had bought herself an identical set, which she now wore. "When you're in the hospital and we look at our bracelets, we'll be thinking about each other," she had said.

"Something new?" asked Paulette, holding my wrist.

I explained to her about the bracelets.

"They were given to you with love, you know."

Again, I slowly nodded. Then Paulette went around to the head of the table and sat on her therapy ball. She was able to hear my abrupt, nervous breathing, I suppose, for she then bent her face close to mine and said, "Now breathe slowly and deeply with me. Come on, we're going to breathe together."

I closed my eyes and with Paulette, took several slow, deep breaths. As I continued to breathe like this, she began to speak in a low, soothing tone – slowly, hypnotically.

"When you enter the operating room, you are going to feel G-d's presence all around. The warm light of G-d's energy will be glowing throughout that room. Each nurse and every doctor is going to have an angel on their shoulders. Everyone in that room is a servant of G-d and is filled with his wisdom. And when you begin to hear the opening notes of the Reiki music, you're going to immediately relax, and your cells are going to feel happy, for you have cellular memory."

Yes, cellular memory. My readings had introduced me to that concept.

"As the music plays, you are going to drift into a deep, long, and restful sleep. And as you sleep, the hand of G-d will be guiding the surgeons' hands as they operate on you and use all their skill flawlessly. G-d will be watching over you the entire time. When the surgeons are done, you are going to wake up and feel well and whole and completely rested, as if you've woken up from the most delicious sleep."

"For a change!" I chimed in.

Paulette rapped my head with a finger.

"Stay with me," she chided, and then continued in her soothing voice.

"You will feel calm and comfortable, and any pain you have will be minimal. Your body will immediately begin to heal from the surgery. Everyone will be amazed at your rapid recovery. During your entire stay in the hospital, you will have a very strong sense of being in the hands of G-d."

And then she did Reiki, silently, sitting at the head of the Reiki table on her therapy ball with my head cradled between her arms, and her hands placed over the chakra of my heart space. I knew why. The heart is the seat of courage.

As I lay in this warm, protective, and deeply comforting cocoon, I felt G-d's presence encompassing the entire room. This is how it must have been as a fetus, back in the womb. Slowly, I began to drift off into a deep sleep.

To end the Reiki session, Paulette placed her palm on my forehead, similar to the way a fairy godmother touches her charges with her magic wand. Startled awake, I settled back into my drug-like Reiki state. Paulette left the room to let me rest for a while.

When Paulette returned to the room, I spoke to her about how calm and protected I was feeling.

"Yes," she said. "It's the feeling of being held and surrounded by mother earth."

Now who was this mythological figure, this mother earth? Certainly I didn't know of her. The only ultimate reality that I knew of was G-d. But I didn't argue the point, for I was feeling totally calmed and just wanted to ride out this state for as long as possible.

Afterward, Mike came back, and we three went down to the concrete deck which overlooked the beach. After we said goodbye to Paulette, Mike and I left her to go down to the sand. We sat at the water's edge, holding hands as we watched the rhythmic waves caress the shore again and again. Do not be afraid, I told Mike, all would be well. Filled with calm, my mind was as unwrinkled by worry as the smooth sand after it is washed and soothed by the timeless ocean.

The hotel suite was pretty nice, with two full beds in the bedroom, a pullout couch in the living room, and a tiny kitchen. We had booked it weeks in advance through Memorial Sloan Kettering. The hotel tower was affiliated with New York Presbyterian Hospital and was only about three short blocks away from Memorial. My hospital stay would be from seven to nine days, and I had packed a small, wheeled suitcase. Mike, Lia, and Zack brought their overnight things in small knapsacks. Zack had wanted to bring his girlfriend, but Mike went ballistic at this suggestion.

"This is not a pleasure trip!" he roared. "Your mother is having major surgery!"

Mike and the kids went out to get some dinner, while I stayed in the hotel suite. My prep, which had consisted of just two little bottles of what tasted like ocean water, had cleaned out my bowels till they were excreting a yellow liquid. Not allowed to have any solid food, I could drink apple juice, and had brought a bottle along to tide me over. The calmness which had settled over me during the Reiki session two days earlier unfortunately had disappeared in this new setting. Damn. The previous night I had slept very well and was fine all day until we had set out in our car for Manhattan. If I could only bring back that calm!

We decided to get to bed early, for we'd have to check into admitting at 6:00 a.m. Mike, who had been nervous all day, was soon asleep. I lay next to him on the narrow bed, watching the clock, for sleep eluded me. The minutes ticked slowly by until four a.m, when Mike, who is blessed with a reliable, internal alarm clock, awoke. Wearily, I got out of bed twenty minutes later to shower. My last normal shower, because the next time I'd be able to bathe, I might have an ileostomy. Since midnight I hadn't had anything to drink. Good thing mine was the first surgery – my mouth wouldn't be so parched. We got ourselves ready, and I said my morning prayers in the tiny kitchen, facing east. Then I woke Zack and Lia, letting them sleep as long as possible.

By 5:30 we were walking in the dark, warm, and muggy morning along York Avenue. In one hand I held my walkman CD player with the Reiki CD and headphones, and I pulled my suitcase along with the other. In no time, we entered the hospital, which was a bright hub of activity, and we checked into pre-admissions. Mike and the kids seated themselves among the quiet tension of the other family members of the soon-to-be patients, while I paced back and forth, full of nervous energy. Before too long, I was called into a small cubicle to identify myself with my hospital and health insurance cards, and my wrist was then strapped with a plastic hospital band.

"Can I have a room with a view of the East River?"

The admissions clerk laughed. "We'll see what we can do."

After about twenty minutes, we were escorted to another waiting room on the sixth floor. Mike and I were called into the pre-op prep area. Zack and Lia had to remain behind in this new waiting room until just before the surgery.

After changing into a hospital gown, a robe, head covering, and blue paper booties, I sat upright on a gurney with Mike by my side. The wait there seemed endless. Between the taking of vitals, I nervously got up and made last minute bathroom stops. I was still excreting yellow liquid. Not to worry, I was told. They'd do a complete rectal flush after I was put under and before the surgery began.

"I'd like to bring my CD and CD walkman with me into the operating room," I informed the nurse.

"We'll give you our own CD player and headphones. For sanitary reasons, we can't allow every patient to take their own CD player into the operating room. But," she added, "I can't guarantee that you'll get your CD back."

Now, that got me agitated. "Well, I'd better get it back! This CD is very important to me. I will be very upset if it gets lost."

The nurse returned with the hospital CD player and headphones, and put a label with my name, hospital ID number, and Dr. Wong's name on my Reiki CD. I settled down a bit.

Finally my escort, a tall fellow clad in light blue scrubs and cap, arrived.

"Can you walk, or do you need a wheelchair?"

Mike laughed. "She goes to the gym every day!"

Zack and Lia were then called in to say goodbye. I gave Lia my Karma bracelets for safekeeping, and we hugged. Then I hugged Zack, who felt tense and distant. Mike walked with me and the escort through a double door and down a hall. Then our escort stopped.

"This is where you stay behind," he said to Mike.

This was it. We stopped, and I handed Mike my watch (he never wore one). We then embraced. Mike gazed down at me and with tears in his eyes called me his "wonderful warrior." I felt like I was going to cry. I didn't want to leave. And anyway, it really wasn't true – me, his "wonderful warrior." It was just that I was pushed and prodded by fate, by circumstance. Letting go of him, I turned and sauntered down the hall with my escort. I took one last look back at Mike. And then we turned a corner.

An electric double door opened to a cool, wide hallway with a domed, sky-blue ceiling with recessed lighting where the slope met the walls. It was quite nice, like the inside of a futuristic spaceship. We then turned left through another set of double doors – the operating room.

Whoa. It was as cold as a butcher's meat locker. A gowned, masked nurse who was arranging a large assortment of operating tools on a draped table greeted me cheerfully. There were several other gowned, masked nurses who were busy checking equipment. How could these people work in this icebox? The anesthesiologist, who was not yet masked, was also cheerful and introduced himself as Dr. Garcia. He explained that in addition to accessing my mediport, he would open an IV line in each arm after I fell asleep. I told Dr. Garcia about my Reiki CD, and he then explained to me that during the surgery, they would all be so busy that they might not think to restart the music. I understood.

A short man with glasses, dressed in light green scrubs, cap, and mask slowly came toward me. He locked his eyes onto mine. Those dark, intense eyes – I had seen them before.

"Dr. Fong!" I fumbled for an appropriate greeting. "How was your trip to London?"

"Oh, I'm glad *that's* over," he laughed.

My goodness, I thought, but I was bleary eyed! An idea entered my head, and I looked at Dr. Fong.

"You *are* a morning person, aren't you?" I asked him.

Dr. Fong chuckled, "Very *much* so!" He was like a kid on his way to an amusement park, eager to get on with the excitement. He was all pumped up.

I didn't see Dr. Wong, but he must have been near. Then, reiterating what Paulette had said to me, I told myself that G-d would be guiding the hands of these doctors.

Dr. Garcia asked me to hop up onto the operating table and lie down. I did so, bringing the CD player and headphones with me, and they soon covered me with a nice, warm blanket. Ahh! After starting the Reiki CD, I began to slowly breathe in and out as the familiar, soothing notes sung out to me, calming me. Bum bum bummm. Bum bum bum bummmm. Yes, you have cellular memory. Repeating to myself all the things that Paulette had told me two days before, I began to go into a state of deep relaxation. Dr. Garcia covered my nose and mouth with a plastic mask, and I soon became extremely drowsy. Then with sudden alarm, I realized that I had forgotten one very important final thing. There was something I needed to say. I had to stay awake for one more moment, for I did not want to fall into that deep sleep without pronouncing those words. As the curtains of consciousness began to close across my mind, I murmured the declaration of faith which has been the last words of my people for a hundred generations: "*Shema Yisroel, Adonai Elohaynu, Adonai Echad.*" Hear, oh, Israel. The Lord is our G-d. The Lord is One.

Then everything went blank.

My Role as a Hospital In-Patient

Gradually, I became aware of the hum of machinery and quiet voices all around me. Back in school, one of our professors had mentioned to us that the sense of hearing is the last sense to leave when consciousness leaves and the first sense to return when consciousness returns. This is quite true. How long I had been lying there, hearing my surroundings, I don't know, but after a while, I realized that I was awake. My eyes opened to a darkened room. Everything was spinning around me as if I were on a merry-go-round. To try to lessen that reeling sensation, I closed my eyes. Then I felt it. There was something jammed down my throat. I began to panic and gag. Somehow, I managed to calm myself and breathe slowly. With eyes still shut, I indicated with my hand at my mouth that I wanted the endotracheal tube taken out.

"Soon."

To make the tube easier to endure, I concentrated on slow breathing. Trying to feel for an ileostomy bag, I touched my abdomen with my hand. Was it there? I didn't feel anything. Then they pulled out the tube, to my relief. But I couldn't take a deep breath, for I was in too much pain.

Mike was there. Why did he look so dark and shadowy? He was just a dark gray outline of himself, and I couldn't see his face. Zack and Lia were there too, both of them hazy gray silhouettes. All of them were spinning, spinning. I heard Mike speak to me.

"Dr. Wong said that the surgery went well, but it was very extensive. It took about eight and half hours, and you were under anesthesia for ten and a half. Dr. Fong did the liver resection. He took out the tumor, and he said that it was bigger than was indicated in the CAT Scan. It was attached to your diaphragm. He also removed your gall bladder because it was inflamed. Dr. Wong did a rectal resection and the temporary ileostomy. He also gave you a complete hysterectomy and took out twenty-four lymph nodes. Seven of them were cancerous."

Unable to keep my eyes open because of the extreme dizziness, I was still mentally lucid. They must have thought that I was sedated, though, because I didn't speak. I couldn't, for I was immobilized and rendered speechless by pain every time I breathed in. Nodding slightly, I listened to Mike tell about how the three of them had sat in the waiting room and gotten periodic updates of the surgery from a nurse. Dr. Fong, in the middle of the surgery, had gotten a call to do an emergency procedure, and had left his fellows to finish up on my liver. Mike and the kids had not eaten all day.

"Would it be okay with you if we went home now and came back tomorrow?"

Yes, I nodded, understanding how exhausted they must have been.

"I'll make sure your suitcase is brought up to your room." And he kissed me on the forehead and left.

The nurses allowed me to moisten my mouth with a lollipop-like sponge which was dipped in ice water. My mouth was so parched that, when no one was looking, I repeatedly dipped the sponge in the water and sucked on it to quench my thirst.

Shortly afterward, two nurses came to sit me up at the edge of the recovery bed so that I could transfer to another bed on which I would be brought to my room. I couldn't even roll onto my side. The pain was unbelievable. The nurses helped me sit up and then stand so that they could put a wide, elastic binder around my abdomen, for support. This, they said, was to make it less painful when I moved. They tugged the binder so that the hole in it was lined up with the ileostomy bag. I was in agony.

"On a scale of one to ten, how much does it hurt?" asked one of the nurses.

"Twenty," I whispered. "It's off the charts."

They brought me to a corner room on the fifteenth floor, with not just a view of the East River and Roosevelt Island, but with wide windows on the southern wall looking out onto the city. They gave me the spot by the East River window, which pleased me. So far, I didn't have a roommate. A nurse then told me that since my surgery had been so extensive, I would not be required to sit up or walk that day. Then they handed me a spirometer. I tried sucking air out of it, but with my excruciating incisional pain, I could only get the indicator up to 500. They wanted me to be able to draw in enough air so that it would reach 2,000. Well, not today. Today I would give in to my pain and exhaustion.

The nurses and aides tended to me with complete compassion. Not only did I have an ileostomy bag, but I also had a bag for the Foley catheter for urine and a J pouch – a small plastic squeeze bag attached to my abdomen by tubing which drained out excess, steak-juice colored fluid which tends to collect around surgical sites. These bags were drained every four hours by the aides. Each of my legs was also encased in a pneumatic sleeve which continually inflated and deflated in order to prevent postsurgical blood clots.

"This button is for your morphine. Whenever you feel you need it for pain relief, just press it," said the nurse, before leaving me alone.

Compulsively, I pressed the button again and again. It was, unfortunately, programmed to respond for only a limited number of times per hour. Click. Click. Click. The morphine IV pump wouldn't react every time, I knew, but I was hopeful.

My room seemed to be cast in a dim, yellow light. Although I didn't know it at the time, the darkness as well as the dizziness was caused by the anesthesia. Since I had forty percent of my liver removed, and it is the liver which removes toxins, it would take several weeks for the anesthesia's effects to completely wear away.

A woman with long black hair entered the room and stood across from the foot of my bed, staring at me. She wore a light blue worker's blouse. Through the dimness and spinning, I strained to read the embroidered words over the front pocket of her shirt. It said "Building Services." The woman began to ask me about my surgery, but as I was in intense pain, I barely responded. Also, I was lucid enough to know that a person from Building Services was not part of my treatment team. Oh G-d, was this going to be a torture scene from a horror movie? When would she leave? She asked me several questions, but

I have learned that in situations like this, the best thing is to be quiet and to just wait. That's what I did. Very wary, I forced myself to keep my eyes open, but I remained silent. After a while, the woman from Building Services stopped talking and became quiet herself. And then, seeing that she would get no answers here, she left. Breathing out in relief, I closed my eyes and then dozed on and off.

Someone was again in the room, I sensed, at the foot of my bed. I opened my eyes, and saw Dr. Wong with one of his fellows, a young doctor whom I hadn't met before. He surprised me – I didn't think that Dr. Wong would come to see me so soon, having spent so much time in surgery with me, but there he was.

"How's your bag?" he asked.

"Which one?" I managed to gasp.

Dr. Wong grinned. He then explained that he had to leave town for a few days, but that his fellows would be taking good care of me. I nodded.

Then I whispered, "Thank you, Dr. Wong, for saving my life."

He nodded and then left with his fellow. For the rest of the night I dozed, in and out of sleep.

The next day, I met three of Dr. Wong's fellows – Dr. Cipriano, Dr. Balsh, and Dr. Hofstetter. The fellows liked to make their hospital rounds early in the morning, starting at about seven o'clock. They were all very nice and good looking, but Dr. Hofstetter's slight German accent unnerved me. I pictured myself as a human experiment in a Nazi concentration camp. Don't be ridiculous, I told myself. The fellows said that they wanted to have a look at my stitches and ileostomy bag. The surgical incision, more than a foot long, had cut through my abs from top to bottom. The stitches, too numerous for me to count in a spinning world, were each spanned by a small clamp. My poor abdomen was now round and swollen, and I looked like a ragged teddy bear which had been repaired with rough stitching.

A transparent ileostomy bag was attached to my abdomen just below and to the right of my belly button. It had a bit of brownish-green liquid in it. Inside the bag, near the top, I could see the cherry red piece of my small intestine which had been turned inside out and sewn to the surrounding skin. It looked like a very ripe miniature tomato. But to me, this, too, was something painful to look at. It was so ugly.

"Your stitches look good and so does the ileostomy," said Dr. Balsh in a slight western twang. He was from Texas, I guessed.

"Do you see the red color of your ileostomy?"

I nodded.

"That means it's healthy," he explained. "If the color should change, you must let the nurses know immediately. That would mean that its blood supply is not getting through."

Now Dr. Hofstetter had his say, in a detectable German accent. "We're going to keep you on clear liquids today. You can have cranberry juice, water, and chicken broth. If you tolerate that well, then tomorrow we'll give you some jelly."

He meant Jello, of course. But I didn't like Jello or jelly, and I stubbornly decided that he could not make me eat either of them. Besides, the very thought of food right then was nauseating. It's incredible how your appetite disappears after abdominal surgery.

"It'll take a few days for your bowels to wake up," said Dr. Balsh, all warm and smiling. "After that, your appetite will slowly return."

They left me to go on to their next patient.

Feeling sorry for myself, I lay there quietly. No longer a normally functioning person with bowel movements, I was now a patient with an artificial device attached to a part of my exposed intestine, and was essentially different from the rest of humanity. The surgeons had altered me physically, and, for the first time since becoming ill, I wondered, "Why me?"

But this sadness only lasted for twenty minutes or so. With scars and all, I was still alive, I reminded myself, and I once again affirmed that everything that G-d did was ultimately for my good. I was determined to make the most of my new circumstance.

An aide came to give me a sponge bath. With her help, I sat up at the edge of the bed after she had set up the basin and towels on the hospital table.

"I can do it myself," I told her.

"Are you sure?"

I nodded. She stayed nearby, in case I should fall, as I slowly and painfully bathed. The point where the J pouch was attached to my abdomen was especially tender and piercing. It was very important not to let that pouch hang, but to pin it up onto a hospital gown, because the weight of it hanging down was extremely painful.

That morning, I coughed up a wad of phlegm, a painful process, as was nose blowing. But I was glad, for I was afraid that, unable to breathe fully and deeply, I would catch pneumonia.

Later on, a nurse and an aide came to help me out of bed so that I could walk. Even with the head of the bed raised, I needed complete help to sit at the edge.

"Would you like us to get you a trapeze?"

Yes, that would help, for my abdominal muscles were useless.

Leaning on a tall rolling walker, with the nurse holding me on one side and the aide dragging along the IV pole on the other, I slowly shuffled forward, eyes half shut as I maneuvered through the spinning hallway, each step an agony to my abdomen. I managed to go around the rectangular path once. As I began the walk, I saw Mike, Lia, and my mother coming down the hall toward me.

"Look, she's walking!" my mother exclaimed. She apparently didn't believe that I'd be able to get out of bed at all.

But it wasn't too long before I had to be helped back into bed. Once around the corridor was all I could manage to do at first. For the remainder of the day, I dozed on and off as Mike tried to engage me in conversation. But it was no use. Before too long I would nod off, succumbing to the residual effects of the anesthesia.

After they left, I asked an aide to help me out of bed so that I could sit on the chair in front of the window. Being upright would be better for my lungs. For hours I sat there, dozing for a few minutes here and there, and staring out at the smokestacks beyond Roosevelt Island when I was awake. The sky was now turning dark, and the red lights near the tops of the stacks winked through the night. My pain was still very intense, much too intense for me to concentrate on doing Reiki to myself. It seemed to get worse at night.

Dr. Fong and Dr. Cantor came in to see me. Dr. Fong pulled up a chair and sat close by. "How are you feeling?"

"Dr. Fong, had I known how painful this recovery would be, I would have never agreed to the surgery. This is just too much."

I meant it. With a liver tumor which was possibly eighty percent dead, I would have taken my chances.

Dr. Fong leaned forward and looked straight into my eyes. He was a good listener. "I know how you must feel–"

"No you don't," I interrupted. "You don't, because I don't think you've ever been on the receiving end of such a surgery."

"That's true. But I do know that each day will get a little better for you," he said sympathetically. "Meanwhile, it's very important that you use the spirometer regularly, despite the pain. And it's also very important that you walk. That's probably the most important thing you can do for yourself."

He handed me the spirometer, and I used all my painful effort to get the ball to rise to 1000. Then he and Dr. Cantor went out to their next patient.

Having grown stiff sitting on the chair with my legs elevated on an ottoman, I asked the aide, Chris, to help me back into bed. He was tall and gentle, and after carefully helping me back, he emptied my bags of their fluids. Then he left.

Earlier that day I had been taken off the morphine pump. They don't keep you on it too long, I suppose because the hospital doesn't want to release a lot of new junkies out onto the city streets. If I asked for it, I could get Percocet for pain.

My abdomen was starting to ache badly. I really needed that Percocet. Where was the call bell? Damn. Chris had forgotten to place it back within my reach. It was tied to the chair by the window. I tried to yell for help, but you need abdominal muscles for that, and mine were useless. I was unable to project my voice.

With my limited mobility, I reached for the in-house telephone on my night table. After managing to grab the receiver, I realized that I didn't know how to make an outside call. The cell phone. It was on the far side of the night table. As I strained to reach it, what came to mind was a scene from an old *Ben Casey* episode, in which a patient, immobilized in an iron lung, and victimized and tortured by a scheming relative, managed to grasp a pencil with his mouth and dial for help on his telephone. That was sort of similar to what was happening now, and I started laughing at myself. Got it. I dialed home.

"Pick up, pick up," I whispered to the cell phone.

Out of a semi-sleep, Mike awoke and answered. Call the nurses' station, I asked him, after explaining the situation, and have them bring me some Percocet. They did, all apologetic.

That night, and every night afterward, I slept clasping my cell phone in my lap.

The morning after Dr. Fong came to speak to me, I slowly got up out of bed by myself and, dragging my IV pole along with the catheter bag hooked to the bottom, I went to get myself towels and washcloths. Determined, I decided to give myself a sponge bath at the bathroom sink, with running water, and then get dressed. Back in school, one of our professors had explained to us that it is much more challenging for patients to perform activities of daily living – bathing, dressing, and toileting – than it is for them to simply ambulate. This was very true, I found. It took a supreme act of will to stand at the sink and methodically wash myself. My abdomen was excruciatingly painful, and I was exhausted to the bone. But later, when I forced myself to walk around the corridors, although that too was painful, it was simply a matter of putting one foot in front of the other and moving forward. That is in fact much easier than standing in one spot and sequencing one's bathing or dressing.

Now I had a roommate, a woman perhaps eight years younger than myself. She too had colon cancer and now had a temporary ileostomy. It was shocking to see a number of young people who were patients. One woman on our floor didn't look older than twenty-five.

When I was done with my sponge bath, I went to my bedside to get dressed. It was very important for me mentally, I knew, to discard the hospital gowns during the day and to wear my own clothes. I despised feeling like a patient, and keeping the hospital gowns on would only intensify those feelings of illness and powerlessness. Under no circumstances would I allow myself to feel that way. I was going to get dressed and feel whole.

When I had done my Level I physical disabilities fieldwork, my supervisor had shown me how to snake a patient's Foley catheter bag through their underwear and pants. Now I put my knowledge to work and snaked the bag through my own underwear and shorts. Tadah! I felt so proud and accomplished. After snaking the catheter bag through, I stood to pull up my underwear and shorts simultaneously, to conserve energy. Energy conservation is an occupational therapy technique taught to people with poor endurance. Shit. I had gotten the underwear backwards. Having exhausted myself from the effort of bathing and dressing, it was just too much work to re-snake the catheter bag out and then back again. I laughed at myself – I'd have to spend the whole day with my underwear wedged up my butt. Alas! Another trial and tribulation!

With my abdomen so painful, I couldn't bend down to get my shoes.

"Would you like some help?" asked the nurse.

"I'll do it." Fishing my toes into a sneaker, I raised my leg up to the edge of the bed so that I could hold my sneaker as I pushed my foot in. After donning both sneakers, I wheeled the IV pole with the attached catheter bag out of the room to the nurse's supply closet to get some tape. Then I taped my CD player to the IV pole, as my pants pockets weren't big enough to hold it. Bocelli – I was listening to him again. Pushing my IV pole contraption in one hand, I was now ready for the day. Lost in the music of Andrea Bocelli, with eyes half shut against the spinning hallway, I forced myself to walk and walk. There were many other patients, dressed in either hospital gowns or their own pajamas, slowly walking the halls as they pushed their IV poles along. I was virtually the only one wearing street clothes.

"You inspire me," said one fellow patient as I passed her in the hall.

"It's all in the music," I answered. "You need some good CDs. That'll help you to walk."

Each day, I walked a little faster and a little longer, and was able to stand a little straighter, despite the pain. But, because my abdominal muscles were now useless, I had to rely more on my back muscles to hold myself upright, and they were aching from the effort. Damn. Instead of putting so much pilates effort toward my abs, I should have concentrated more on strengthening my lower back. Next time I'd know better.

My friend, Marlene, called me later that day, saying she was going to come and visit.

"What should I bring you?"

I didn't need anything, and I told her so.

"No, really. I want to get you something. Would you like a nightgown?"

No, because at night, I was sweating profusely. My body was gradually ridding itself of the excess fluid which it had retained because of the anesthesia. It was much more practical for me to wear hospital gowns at night and discard them the next morning.

"How about a book?"

Was she kidding? I couldn't even focus my eyes enough to watch television, let alone read.

"Flowers?"

Now why would I want that?

"Really, Ruth, I want to get you something."

She was really insistent. I caved in. "Get me a Bocelli CD."

"Which one?"

I told her the name of the one which I already owned.

The next day, she came, and brought me a fantastic CD, which I would play over and over again as I walked the halls. It was a great, inspiring gift.

Because I was walking for so long, the nighttime pneumatic leg sleeves were discharged. My roommate wanted to know why I no longer had to wear them at night, whereas she still did.

"Mrs. Levine walks for miles," explained the nurse.

Now I was able to eat some solid food, which I did unenthusiastically. The kosher food which I was able to order was pre-cooked and largely unappetizing. What's more, every one of us patients who had a new ileostomy had to be on a "low residue" diet for a month, and that consisted of low fat and low fiber. The only fresh fruits we were allowed to have were bananas; other fruits consisted of canned peaches or apple sauce. Real hospital fare. I picked at my food. Mike would often finish whatever I had left on my plate. Dr. Balsh came in once after lunch and took note of how much I had eaten.

"You've eaten about half of your food. That's very good – much more than I would have expected."

"Listen," I told him. "I've got a husband here who'll eat nearly anything you put in front of him. If I really wanted to fool you, I'd have him eat all of my lunch. You'd never know."

The food was dreadful, but thankfully, my mother brought plastic tubs filled with her chicken soup and pieces of chicken and vegetables. In the evenings, I'd warm up a little bit of it in the microwave in the service area and have that before going around the halls for my evening walk.

The intense pain was subsiding a bit. Now I was able to do Reiki to myself, concentrating on my very tender abdomen. During one such evening session, as I lay with my eyes closed, listening to my Reiki CD, I again sensed someone standing at the foot of my bed. It was Dr. Fong and Dr. Cantor. Hurriedly, I turned off the CD and took off my headphones. They were glad to see that I was feeling a little better.

"I know how upset you were the other evening when I came to see you," began Dr. Fong. Apparently, he had been troubled by my reaction to the painful after effects of the surgery – troubled enough to make another bedside visit.

"But I want you to keep in mind," he continued, "that in no other hospital could you have three surgeries in one as you've had here. Any place else you'd have to go through three separate surgeries – and three separate recoveries!"

Could you imagine – going through all that again and again?

"I'd slit my wrists!" I declared.

Now that the pain was not so intense, I was able to think more clearly. After the doctors left, the realization slowly grew in me that I was indeed fortunate, and that these doctors had done an incredible thing for me. Two teams of doctors had stood over me for eight and a half hours and had used all their skill and knowledge so that I could live. For them, it was just part of their daily routine. But for me, it was nothing short of remarkable. Those doctors were my heroes.

From then on, I was more careful to orient my underwear carefully when I got dressed. I didn't make the same mistake with the catheter bag again. And with my wonderful CDs, despite the extreme fatigue and the sharp incisional pain, I was soon able to walk for more than an hour at a time. And as I walked to the music, I held before myself, in my mind's eye, the self-image which I had created with Karla's guidance. I was walking towards that healthy, whole person whom I longed to be.

After the doctors came on their morning rounds, I got into a routine of washing, dressing and then walking around and around the corridor for at least an hour in the morning and again in the afternoon. In the evening, after visiting friends and relatives left, and after changing into a hospital gown, I'd go for one last walk.

Like stars across the sky
We were born to shine
All of us here
Because we believe.

Bocelli was cheering me on. To ward off my spinning surroundings, I was still in the habit of walking with my eyes half shut. As I rounded the corner of the corridor one evening, pushing my IV pole along, I nearly collided into Dr. Fong and Dr. White. They were surprised to see me. Dr. White looked especially proud of my walking ability, as if she herself had guided me through my first baby steps. These doctors seemed to get a great deal of pleasure from seeing their patients' progress.

"Try to straighten up when you walk," advised Dr. Fong. It was true. I and many of the other patients who had similar operations were slumped over from the pain of the abdominal incision.

To demonstrate, Dr. Fong stood tall and took in a deep breath.

"This way, your lungs will fill up more fully and your organs will have more room. It will aid in your recovery."

Standing straight – that was so hard to do. It was painful. But I became mindful of it, and from then on tried to keep my back straight whenever I walked. It would be several months before I'd be able to do so without having to make a conscious effort to hold myself upright.

Before too long, one of Dr. Wong's fellows – Dr. Ojibwe – came during morning rounds to remove the J pouch.

"Have you ever removed a J pouch before?" I asked her. I didn't want any novices futzing around with me.

"Several times," she answered.

"On a scale of one to ten," I asked, "how much will it hurt?"

"Oh, about a three."

Huh. They always understate your pain. "Then I take that to be a nine," I concluded.

She grasped the plastic tubing of the pouch close to my abdomen and gave a firm yank. G-d! It felt like she shoved a lit sparkler into me.

"Are you all right?" she asked. I was panting from the pain.

Nodding, I gasped. "I was right. It was a nine."

The smell of tomato sauce wafted up to my nose as I was taking my morning sponge bath at the sink. That was odd. The previous evening, I had eaten some chicken with potatoes and tomato sauce. I looked down, and to my horror saw a stream of what looked like paté leaking out from under the wafer tape of my ileostomy pouch. Oh no! I called for help, but Jen, my nurse that day, couldn't come right away. With the extra wash cloth which I had brought with me, I sopped up the leaking feces, then threw my bathrobe over my shoulders and went to lie down in bed to wait for Jen. One's small intestines are comprised of involuntary muscle, and you don't have any ability to stop the flow of digested food through them. The feces just kept coming out in small, unexpected spurts.

She finally came, and together, step by step, with me verbalizing every move, we changed the wafer together. The trick to changing the wafer – the rubber "gasket" which surrounds the ileostomy and is attached to the surrounding skin with its own adhesive – is to do it before breakfast, on an empty stomach, to prepare all your materials before you actually need to apply them, and to work fast. Unfortunately, I had already had my breakfast, but with our four hands, Jen and I were able to clean the surrounding skin and neatly apply a fresh wafer and snap an ileostomy bag onto it. Although I was supposed to keep the wafer on for at least three days, I decided the following morning to change it again all by myself, just to prove that I could. I was successful.

What I was not so successful at was urinating. Five days after my surgery, the catheter was removed. I went to the recreation room to email a former classmate, but my bladder began to feel extremely distended. By the time I hobbled back to my bed, I was in agony. I was simply unable to pass any urine. Nothing which I had experienced thus far was as painful and frightening as this feeling of a bursting bladder which couldn't be emptied. The nurse performed an ultrasound of my bladder to check for urine retention. It was full, all right. She attempted, painfully, to reinsert the Foley catheter, and did so on the second try.

"The nerves to your bladder were probably irritated during the surgery," explained Dr. Wong the next morning. He had returned from his trip, and was now making the morning rounds with his fellows.

"You had a slight amount of bleeding during the surgery, and that has affected the nerves to your bladder. In time, things should start working more normally."

In less than a week after the surgery, even though I was still hooked up to IV fluids via my mediport, I was allowed to shower in the bathroom in my hospital room. That required a bit of careful planning, as you had to be careful not to dislodge any of the tubing. I ran the water as hot as I could and kept the IV pole, which I now used as a towel rack, close to the small corner shower stall so that I'd have plenty of slack in the lines. Ah! One of life's greatest pleasures is to take a hot shower and get completely clean!

As I pushed aside the plastic curtain to step out of the stall, the bathroom door flew open. It was the janitor, who had come to empty the trash. He took a look at the tubes which sprouted from me like wild vines and at my distended abdomen with the ileostomy bag and the long line of skeletal-like clamps, and gasped.

"Why don't you knock?!" I roared.

He scampered out. I looked so grotesque that I had scared the hell out of him. As Mike was to later note, it was "like a reverse *Psycho.*"

That day, my IV line was discharged and my catheter was removed for the second time. My aide, Stephanie, set me up in the bathroom with soft lighting and with the warm water of the shower tinkling against the tile of the stall to create the proper ambiance for peeing. To help me relax, I had brought my Reiki CD in with me. But I had to bear down painfully on my tender abs and only managed to urinate a tiny trickle each time I tried. My bladder became more and more filled, and the discomfort once again turned into intense pain.

My nurse for the evening, Lisa, came with an "assistant" – another young nurse – to reinsert the catheter. Soon, I realized that she needed an assistant because she was inexperienced. Her attempts were agonizing.

"Get another nurse," I demanded.

She consulted with her assistant, and they summoned an older, more skilled nurse, who did the job quickly and painlessly. In no time, my catheter bag was filled.

"They've got to get that catheter out of you," said Debbie. Her mother, who was very familiar with such things, having been hospitalized several times, had told her that the catheter would only lead to problems for me down the road. But what was I to do? Without it, I couldn't urinate sufficiently. It would just have to remain in for the time being.

That night, I vomited three times, and I noticed that in place of fluid or mushy feces, my ileostomy bag was largely blown up with gas. By now, I had been emptying it myself into the toilet. By the morning, my "output" had slowed to a mere trickle, and there wasn't much to dump out.

Risa came to visit me that day, and entertained me with her numerous stories. Unfortunately, during her visit, I again vomited copiously into a bucket. The nurses were aware, and they sent a good looking resident with a French accent to examine me. He was from Montreal. To make them more human to me, I was always asking those doctors about themselves. He said that it often happens that ileostomies can stop working for a while during the recovery period, and he mentioned the possibility of giving me a naso-gastric tube, which I dreaded. My roommate, who had been vomiting profusely, now had an NG tube, and she said it was extremely uncomfortable. The resident then said that he'd first try eliminating all solid food.

"Just drink sips of water."

Then he had nursing reinsert an IV line so that I'd have more fluids.

"We'll also take an x-ray of your abdomen to rule out a blockage."

After Risa left, a young guy from patient escort came with a wheelchair to take me to the radiology department in the basement for an x-ray. With my IV bag hanging from an attached pole and my catheter bag hooked underneath the chair, we went down in the elevator and navigated the twisting hallways to radiology. Everything was a long wait. My escort left me in the hall, seated in the wheelchair, to wait among an assorted group of debilitated patients until it was my turn to be x-rayed.

After the x-ray, there was another long wait in the hallway. Where the hell was my escort? I wanted to return to my room, go for an afternoon walk, and then rest in bed. But there I was, stuck waiting. I peered up and down the hall and glanced over at the little office which was recessed behind a waist high partition in the wall. The people there were busy booking appointments and answering phones and were oblivious to me. Hmmm, I thought. Let's see. What would happen if . . .

Looking left and right to make sure that nobody was paying any attention, I slowly wheeled myself down the hall. Having been down this way only once, I had a vague recollection of how to get back to the elevators. A sign then pointed right, and I followed it to another long hallway, now going at a fast clip in order to put lots of distance between me and the radiology department.

From far behind, I heard the sound of fast-paced walking. Without looking back, I began to wheel the chair at high speed, using big long strokes. The distant footsteps now sped up, and I heard someone huffing and puffing. The running strides sounded closer as I neared the elevator bank. A scene from a movie flashed before my eyes: *The Great Escape* with Steve McQueen on his motorcycle, trying to escape the Germans and leaping the barbed wire. Finally, my pursuer, breathing heavily, caught up to me.

"What's your last name?" he asked, all out of breath as he jogged beside me. I looked up. It was one of the people from the radiology office.

"Levine."

Without breaking his stride, he roughly grabbed the handles of the wheelchair.

"Where are you going?" he demanded, angry, and gasping for air.

"The M elevators."

He started to wheel me to the elevators. With a sly smile, I looked up at my captor.

"You sound out of breath," I remarked with feigned nonchalance, rather pleased that he, the healthy one, was winded, whereas I, the cancer patient, was not. Had I been able to use my leg muscles, I mused, instead of my smaller arm muscles to propel the chair, he would have never caught up with me.

"I'm a big, old, out-of-shape, fat guy who needs to go to the gym!" he spewed angrily between huffs for air.

Still fuming, he brought me to my room. Casually, I hooked my IV and catheter bags back onto my IV pole, and he stormed off with the wheelchair.

"That's something your father would have done!" laughed Mike. He had come with Rhonda and Elliot shortly after I had been returned to my room. We spent the rest of the afternoon listening to Elliot's funny hospital stories. Before long, they were gone, and for the remainder of the day I sat staring out at the silent smokestacks beyond my window, as they winked through the gray evening light.

Lia had a sore throat and had been staying at home. We spoke by cell phone, though, every day.

"I miss you," she now lamented. "When are you coming home?"

I couldn't really answer that. I had to go home functional, ileostomy and all.

"Look out the window at the moon," I told her. The dark clouds in the sky were starting to break up. "Do you see it?"

"Mmm hmm."

"Just think. Right now, even though we're miles away, you and I are both looking at the same thing – at the moon. If you think about that, then maybe it won't seem that we're so far apart."

"I still want you to come home."

I wanted that too. I longed to go home.

Because my ileostomy had stopped working, my hospital discharge was put on hold. A new fellow, a young blonde doctor with a Canadian accent, came to examine me the next morning.

"Are you from Montreal?" I asked, as she palpated my abdomen.

"No, Toronto."

Dr. Toronto looked down at me doubtfully. "I may have to put an NG tube in you," she said authoritatively. "Your abdomen is rather distended. You're a slim woman, and I would think that it's not like this normally. We'll have to keep a close eye on it."

I dreaded the prospect of having an NG tube. This, too, I had a sense, was something which I was supposed to experience. Fortunately for me, I got a reprieve, as my ileostomy slowly began to function again. Now I was assigned the job of measuring and recording how much waste I was excreting. That wasn't a problem, because they gave each of us ostomy patients a translucent pitcher with measurement lines on the side into which we emptied the contents of our bags before dumping it into the toilet. After a day of normal ileostomy functioning, Dr. Balsh decided that I could go home.

Unfortunately, on the day I was to be discharged, I awoke with a fever of 102, and Dr. Balsh again postponed my discharge. Happily for me, Dr. Ojibwe came that morning to remove the clamps from my stitches. She worked very carefully and gently, and it didn't hurt at all.

I was now starting to feel extremely ill, for like many adults, I find fever to be very debilitating. Feeling too sickly to go for a walk, I spent the day in bed. A technician from the lab came to draw blood in order to find out why I was running the fever.

Later in the day, another young man from patient escort came with a wheelchair to bring me down to radiology for a CAT scan. They wanted to check for any infected fluid retention. He hung the catheter bag under the chair. This time, I wasn't hooked up to an IV, as that had been disconnected from my mediport the previous day.

"I'm so cold," I told the escort.

He grabbed a blanket from my bed and draped it around my shoulders. Then we were off.

Again, I had another very long wait down in the hall by the radiology department. Finally, I was taken in for the CAT scan, the results of which were normal. They didn't see any infected fluid.

Now I was back in the wheelchair, waiting for my escort to come and return me to my room. How I wanted to just lie covered up in bed! But like all patients, I had to wait.

Well, I didn't want to wait. Why should I? So, once again, I unobtrusively surveyed my surroundings. This time, I quietly got up from the wheelchair and hooked the catheter bag to the cargo pocket on the side of my shorts. After adjusting the blanket like a shawl around my shoulders, I walked off.

When I got back to my room, my nurse for the day, Diane, told me that they were frantic down in radiology. There was a missing patient – me. We both had a good laugh over the havoc I was causing.

Still feverish, I went to bed and stayed there for the next two days. Mike was not able to come to the hospital as frequently as before, for school had resumed and he had to be back at work. But my Uncle Myer and Aunt Millie came by to check in on me.

The worst part of the fever was the wracking chills which took hold of me the first night. The nurse smacked a couple of disposable hot packs against the window sill to activate them and tucked them under my pile of blankets to warm me up. It seemed to take forever for the chills to subside.

The next morning, with great effort, I got washed and dressed, only to flop back into bed for the remainder of the day. That evening,

I did something I hadn't done in a while – I pressed my call bell and asked for help.

"Chris," I whispered weakly, when the aide came to my bedside, "I need your help. I'm too sick to get out of bed." I explained to him where to find my container of chicken soup in the service kitchen refrigerator, and gave him instructions on how to warm it up. I would subsist on the soup and hot tea.

The fever was draining me, and I didn't have the energy to change into a hospital gown that night. Even the thought of re-snaking the catheter bag out of my pants was exhausting, so I slept in my clothes.

That morning, I woke up drenched in sweat. Jen was again my nurse. She hadn't seen me since the previous week and was surprised that I was still there. Patients who have ileostomy surgery usually stay in the hospital from seven to nine days. I was now there for eleven.

"You'll feel better if you shower. Come on, get your butt into gear."

Shivering, I took a hot shower, then dressed in fresh hospital gowns and went back to my bed, only to be disturbed by the technician who was now coming every morning to draw blood from my mediport in search for the cause of my fever.

My nurse had given me a small supply of disposable hot packs which you activated by twisting as if you were wringing out a wash cloth. They were good for fever chills and even for post-operative pain, which I still had. But some of them were difficult to twist open. In the evening, I ventured out of bed and walked over to the nurse's station. I was looking for a man. Any man. Peering through the glass, I caught sight of a doctor (he was the only one at the station wearing a lab coat). I tapped on the glass until he looked up at me. Then I motioned to him with my crooked index finger. Alarmed, he pointed to himself. I nodded and kept beckoning with my index finger. He came over to the window.

"Do you want me for something?" he asked warily. The nurses and secretaries all stopped to watch what looked like an incident in the making.

"Yes. You look like a strong guy." I held up the hot pack for him to see. "Can you open this for me?"

He looked relieved that that was all I wanted. The nurses all smirked in amusement, and even more so as the doctor unsuccessfully struggled to twist open the hot pack. Finally the receptionist took it from him, gave it a strong twist, and returned it to me through the window slot. I thanked her and happily walked back to bed with my little bag of comfort.

The next morning, I woke up without fever and was ravenous. Dr. Balsh came early on morning rounds.

"We're pretty sure now about the cause of your fever. It was a UTI which spilled over into your blood."

I was resigned for the worst. "Sepsis," I said quietly. A blood infection. Often fatal.

"No, it didn't get that far yet. We're putting you on IV antibiotics to make sure that it doesn't. When you go home, you may have to go home with IV antibiotics, too. And there's still the possibility that your mediport has become infected. These infections like to lodge in foreign bodies like mediports. If it's infected, it'll have to come out."

"Will I have to go back into surgery for that?" I asked.

"No, no. It's a minor procedure to remove it. You won't need any anesthesia. We have an examination room on this floor; I can do it there with a nurse to assist me."

Shortly after he left, a technician came to draw more blood from my mediport. Now feeling paranoid about the spread of infection, I asked him to don a surgical mask. I certainly didn't want any more bacteria to find their way into my bloodstream.

Later that morning, I stood at the window facing the East River, saying the morning prayers. It was odd, looking out that window at the street below and the river beyond. One heard no noise from the outside. The windows did not open, and they were sound proof. It was like watching a silent movie.

As I stood there, reciting my prayers and gazing onto the silent scene below, two men in lab coats entered the room and stood near my bed. They respectfully waited until I was done. One of them, a thirty-ish looking man with dark hair and an Israeli accent, introduced himself as Daniel. I didn't catch the other fellow's name, if he even did mention it. They were from the Department of Infectious Diseases. Daniel was obviously the experienced one, and the other guy was there to learn from him. That's how things are often done in a teaching hospital. Daniel started asking me a series of questions – my age, occupation, address – like a detective.

"Do you have any pets?"

That was an odd question from an investigator from Infectious Diseases.

"Yes. I have two cats."

"What are their names?"

I became exasperated.

"Why are you asking me all this nonsense? To see if I'm sane?" As if he could verify the information! It then occurred to me that a urinary tract infection can cause temporary symptoms of dementia, and he could have been checking for that. He was apparently satisfied that I was alert and oriented, and he proceeded to give me a thorough physical examination. He reiterated what Dr. Balsh had told me earlier about the UTI which had spilled over into my blood, possibly infecting my mediport, and said he would come back again.

That day, Dr. Balsh returned to remove my Foley catheter for the third time – and hurray! – I was able to urinate. The nurse put a "hat" – a plastic measuring cup fitted around the toilet rim and suspended over the bowl – in the toilet, so they could measure how much I was urinating. It was 400 cc's – not bad – and, thankfully, after checking with a catheter, the nurse announced that there was no residual urine in my bladder. Nevertheless, I still had to bear down painfully on my abdominals, and the sensation of having to urinate was missing. Now I knew I had to pee when there was a vague, painful pressure in my pelvic area.

Feeling much better, I was back to walking the hallway again, but now, as I no longer had a catheter bag or a continuous IV infusion (although an IV shunt had been inserted in my arm for my periodic antibiotic treatment), I was no longer tethered to an IV pole onto which I could tape my CD player.

"You could take a pole along with you, if you like," suggested Jen, the nurse.

"Oh, no," I answered. "That IV pole is a symbol of illness, and I want nothing to do with it." It was a milestone for me to be rid of it.

When Dr. Balsh came by early the next morning, I asked him about the pathology reports from my surgery. It had taken all this time for the pathologists to thoroughly examine the tumors and write up their findings.

"The report came back, and it shows that eighty percent of the liver tumor was definitely dead and the rectal tumor was ninety percent dead. And the margins were all clean. That's great news."

He was smiling broadly, mirroring the elation which was welling up within me.

"But," he continued, "I'm pretty sure you'll have to go back on follow-up chemo for four months, because of those seven cancerous lymph nodes we removed. After a recovery period from the chemo, you can have your ileostomy reversed." He paused, and I let all that sink in.

"It also looks like your mediport is infected. So, I'll be back sometime later today, and we'll get that done."

He left, and I lay there with my thoughts tumbling through my head. Those tumors, after five cycles of chemo, had been mostly dead. Yes! It had to have been so, else, how could I have done all that I did in the gym? But now, I faced the prospect of going through yet more chemo. In resignation, I sighed. It wasn't over yet. I had to make myself view the upcoming chemo positively. I decided to think of it as the light at the end of the tunnel – at the end of which lay the ultimate, although often under-appreciated, gift from G-d: freedom in the form of good health.

After my morning shower, I lay on my bed, in my street clothes, with my pants pulled down below my hips. All my ostomy supplies were at hand and I was changing the wafer.

"Mrs. Levine?"

I recognized the accented voice from behind my bed curtain.

"Come, in," I told Daniel, the detective from Infectious Diseases.

With all of my visual attention focused on the task at hand, I was working fast and efficiently, trying to keep one step ahead of any feces which might spurt out of my ileostomy. Out of the corner of my eye, I caught Daniel's fascinated stare.

"I have to look at what I'm doing, but I'm listening to you. Speak."

"The plan is this," he said, his eyes riveted to my abdomen. "We're going to continue taking blood cultures. If they're negative, we'll send you home without an IV but with antibiotics in pill form. If they're not negative, we'll see."

Pressing the wafer firmly around the ileostomy, I gave him the thumbs up sign.

"Super! And Dr. Balsh said that he's going to remove my mediport today."

Daniel gave a brief nod, then left.

By the afternoon, I was starting to feel feverish again. Where was that Dr. Balsh? Shouldn't he have come to take out my mediport by now?

Where could he be, I asked one of the nurse practitioners.

"Dr. Balsh is down in the OR."

By six p.m. I was tired and feeling very ill. Had Dr. Balsh forgotten about me? Beside myself, I marched myself down to the nurses' station.

"Where's Dr. Balsh?"

The receptionist looked up from her paperwork.

"He's down on the sixth floor." That's where the operating rooms were.

"You tell Dr. Balsh," I began aggressively, then stopped myself and thought about what I would say. I have a bad habit of blurting out my thoughts. Not wanting to sound too overbearing, nor wanting to sound like I was giving orders, I would have to modulate my words.

"Tell Dr. Balsh that Mrs. Levine said" – now, that was better, I would not be putting words into their mouths, and they could blame me for the message – "to get his fat ass up to the fifteenth floor and take out this frickin' mediport!"

I pulled the neck of my shirt below my collar bone so she could see what I was referring to.

As if I had an angel sitting on one shoulder, opposite the devil who surely sat on the other, I heard an internal voice chide me, "Be polite!"

"Please," I added, heeding my better angel.

"Shall I write that in bold?" asked the receptionist, with equal parts of annoyance and boredom.

"Absolutely!" I insisted, letting my fever stoke my devil's fire.

Later that evening, I was lying in my bed, feverish and hoping to nod off to sleep, when Dr. Balsh appeared in my room, dressed in green scrubs and cap. He had obviously been in the operating room the entire day.

"Dr. Balsh," I greeted him dryly, "overworked and underpaid."

He nodded tiredly in agreement.

"Let's get that mediport out of you."

"Are we going to the examination room?"

"No, we can do it here as you lie in bed."

"Don't you need a nurse to help you?" I asked, doubtfully.

"That's not necessary. It's a very minor procedure. If we were putting it in then we'd need an operating room."

He had me sign a consent form and then proceeded to prepare for minor surgery. Raising the height of the bed and hospital tray, he then draped them carefully, like a house painter covering the floors with drop cloths. After having me pull my hospital gown below the mediport, he draped me, too. Most of the surgical prep consisted of this extensive draping. Then Dr. Balsh washed and gloved his hands, donned a mask, and unwrapped his surgical tools from their cloth covering. He neatly laid them out on the hospital table, then washed the skin over and around the mediport with a surgical soap solution.

"You'll just feel the needle when it first goes in. After that, the lidocaine will numb you up."

I didn't even try to look down at where he injected me. Through everything I had experienced, I was able to endure it all as long as I didn't look. Never could I bear the sight of needles piercing my skin – not even for simple blood work.

Dr. Balsh was now using his scalpel, I knew, because he was sponging away blood.

"You must be very handy at home," I told him, seeing the correlation between surgical work and tasks requiring planning and dexterity.

Dr. Balsh nodded. "I also enjoy woodworking."

As he slowly disconnected the mediport tubings from their vascular attachments, I felt a terrible tugging. It seemed to take forever.

"Come on, come on, Balsh," I whispered, gritting my teeth through my discomfort. "You can do it."

One last tug. He held up the bloody mediport with what looked like a pair of nose pliers. It resembled a small, round, metal and plastic electronic speaker with a narrow, white, rubber tube attached to one side.

"Can I have it?" I asked.

"What, this? Why?"

"I want it as a souvenir to always remember what I've gone through."

He understood. "Of course. Let me just snip off a bit of the tubing. We'll send it down to pathology just to confirm that it was infected. And I'll stitch you up. I also enjoy sewing."

"Dr. Balsh," I said, as he began to close up the wound, "don't ever be on the other side of those surgical tools."

Only four or five stitches, and he was done. Now I would be free of that fever. And the mediport – that symbol of extreme illness – would no longer be imbedded in me, but would go into my dresser drawer at home, to be taken out from time to time like a relic in a new religious ritual, whose purpose is to remember the past – and relive it in one's heart – in order to be grateful for the present.

Finally, two days later, I was scheduled to be discharged. Dr. Balsh had come by the morning after he removed the mediport, to see how I was doing. The site was very sore, but I now had no fever and was feeling so much better. He wouldn't be in the next day – the day I was to go home.

"Remember not to lift anything heavier than twenty pounds. And if you do go back to the gym, keep the elliptical on a low resistance so as not to strain the stitches. They'll be at their strongest about two months after the surgery."

That was six weeks from now. I had frozen my gym membership till then. Good thing. If I couldn't use the elliptical at a high resistance level, I might as well just walk.

"Stay well," he continued, "and we'll see you in the clinic in about two months." And then, with a smile, Dr. Balsh added, "Try to behave yourself." Previously, I had boasted to him about my exploits of escaping from the radiology department.

"I'll try," I answered, smiling and shaking my head, "but it won't do any good."

A Crash Course in Pain

The day of my discharge arrived. Mike, Gary, and my mother were scheduled to come by at about 11:00 a.m., when I would sign out. Until then, I'd have time to take one last walk around the corridor. During breakfast, Dr. Toronto came by with a posse of residents and one big wig doctor who wasn't even wearing a collared shirt or a lab coat. Instead, he wore a cable knit sweater. I didn't catch his name, but it was obvious that he was the senior doctor. I was reminded of movies of World War II, where the high ranking officer, usually British, often took the liberty of wearing some civilian garb, just to demonstrate how above regulations he was. Dr. Sweater let Dr. Toronto do all the talking.

"Look, she's dressed!" exclaimed Dr. Toronto.

Well, duh, I'd been getting dressed since the second day after my surgery.

"How has your ileostomy been working?"

It was working fine, I told her.

She felt my abdomen, which was now considerably flatter than when she had first come in to see me.

"No abdominal pain?"

"Just from the incision."

I wondered if she was disappointed that she didn't get to put an NG tube down my nose and throat. Clearly, I had dodged that bullet.

After the troop of doctors left, I got up to walk around the hall, listening to my music as I went at a fast clip. The troop was moving down the hall to other patients' rooms, and I kept passing them again and again, inwardly delighted that I could literally walk circles around them.

The nurses generously gave me two shopping bags full of ileostomy supplies, which would last for at least two weeks, until I could receive more after placing an order with a surgical supply company. And then, after signing the discharge papers and receiving the bottles of my oral antibiotic and the diuretic which would prevent fluid from accumulating around my still regenerating liver, we left. I had been in the hospital a total of fifteen days.

As we rode in Gary's car, I was entranced by the scenes of life which played out before us on the city streets. All the sights, noises, and smells! After more than two weeks of merely observing the ostensibly silent scene of York Avenue and the East River from fifteen floors up, I was seeing it all up close. Now it came alive with all five of my senses taking everything in.

As we finally reached the Turnpike, Mike turned to me and asked, "So how does the armpit of New Jersey look?"

"It looks great," I replied. And to me, it did.

As we approached home, I was fascinated to see that the new shopping plaza near our development, for which the land had been leveled, was now starting to take shape. As we sped by, I twisted in my seat and gazed at it like a wide-eyed toddler.

Finally, we arrived home. Zack was at work, but Lia was there waiting, and we gave each other a big hug. Then I cried in relief that I was back. The whole experience of leaving the hospital and re-entering the world had been very intense, and I was exhausted.

That evening, as the sun slowly turned orange-gold low in the sky, I was happy to just sit in the living room with my family. I looked out at the grass and trees as a soft breeze blowing through the patio screen door carried the sweet chirps of the birds and tree frogs. It was a delight to sit there, breathing in the beauty of it all.

"I'm applying for the nursing program at school," Zack informed me.

That was surprising to me, for I didn't think he was suited for the nursing profession. He was such a good bullshit artist that he ought to be a salesman, I thought.

Did he know what he was getting into?

"Come here," I said as I walked over to him, "I want to show you something."

Pulling my pants slightly below my hips, I revealed my transparent ileostomy bag. The cherry red piece of small intestine was clearly visible.

"If you become a nurse," I explained, "you'll have to look at stuff like this. And you'll have to handle stuff like this, too." And do it compassionately.

Zack shrugged. "That doesn't bother me."

Oh, well, I tried to set him straight. To no avail.

It was extremely difficult to lie down flat, for I didn't have a hospital bed on which the head could be raised, nor did I have a trapeze. And I woke up in the middle of the night a bit confused. "Huh!" I said to myself in disgust, "they don't even bother to check your vitals in this place!" It was only after I had lain awake for a few minutes that I realized that I was not in yet another hospital, but was back home.

The next morning, before going on to work, Mike drove to my mother's home to pick her up. She had insisted on staying with me during the day; Zack and Lia were now at school, and she didn't want me to be alone. But, as I was accustomed to doing things for myself and because I couldn't see the justice in having my eighty-nine-year-old mother do tasks around my house, she spent the time in our home either chatting with me, reading the newspaper, or dozing off. I was quite capable of washing a dish after I ate. As for more demanding chores, well, they could wait till I felt better.

After my morning prayers, I ate my meager breakfast. It would take several weeks for my appetite to return; having to remain on the bland, low-residue diet for the next month didn't help it any. Then I showered, got dressed, and told my mother that I was going out for a walk.

"I'll go with you," she said. "I don't want you to go alone."

"I'm perfectly able to walk. I did it all the time in the hospital."

"But you're still dizzy!" she insisted. "You might fall."

"I won't fall. And even though I've had surgery, I can still walk a lot faster than you. You won't be able to keep up."

She saw that she'd get nowhere. "Well, take your cell phone with you. And turn it on."

With the cell phone now in my pocket and a bottle of water in one hand, I headed out the door.

"Don't run!" she called after me.

I laughed. As if I could!

As I walked along the cul-de-sacs of my development, I marveled at the various shapes of leaves and the subtle green shadings of everything that grew. What a beautiful, shining world! And I was back to enjoy it again.

Walking outside was harder than it had been in the hospital. The sidewalk was rough and less forgiving on my incision, as were the sidewalk curbs. To baby my sore abdomen, I slowed down. And I sipped lots of water, for now that my large intestine was bypassed, my body wasn't reabsorbing the water in my intestinal tract and I could easily become dehydrated. Dr. Balsh had warned me about that.

My cell phone rang.

"Where are you?" It was my mother.

"In Gary's section." My brother lived on the other side of our development.

"Are you coming home?"

This question struck me as rather funny.

"Well, yeah. I'm not planning on running away."

She didn't see the humor. "I want you to come home now."

"I'll be home soon."

I closed my cell phone and continued on my way, finishing my walk. My mother had reverted to treating me like a five year old. Only, when I was five, instead of telling me to come home, she would have told me to go back outside!

For the next two weeks I was unable to drive, for hitting the brake pedal can put stress on the abs and on any incision there. During this time, I was a virtual prisoner of my neighborhood. But I was soon to become a virtual prisoner of my home. My ileostomy wafer started to leak.

This had happened only once in the hospital, and since then I had felt that I had it under control. I had even declined a home visit from an ostomy nurse. Now, only a few days after returning home, I found myself changing the wafer sometimes two or three times a day. It was very discouraging.

Mike was disgusted with me.

"Why couldn't you have made that appointment?"

"I thought that everything was okay. I had no problems in the hospital." It was true.

He didn't buy that. "You're stubborn. You're just like your father. You think you can do everything! You're arrogant!"

I was too upset to refute him. Besides, if he saw that, then there must at least be some truth to it.

Now, whenever I went out for a walk, I would carefully stuff paper towels around the wafer to absorb any leakage. A sudden leakage was my constant concern. And a situation such as this can sharply curtail one's social life, to say the least.

Well, that Saturday night, Rhonda and Risa came by to pick me up and bring me by car to Rhonda's house. She was having a little gathering of friends. Risa had the crazy idea of setting up Rhonda's oldest son with the daughter of one of their mutual friends; both young people had never been on a date before. Now they would be on a non-pressured mock date in Rhonda's house as the rest of us chatted and ate the goodies which Rhonda had bought.

She had gotten kosher chicken and kugel for me, but my appetite was still stunted, and I picked at the food. Feeling bone-weary, I still had fun listening to everyone's amusing stories.

After eating, we moved to the living room, my friends sitting on the large sectional and I off to the side on an easy chair. Then it hit me. Just as I was now separated from them by this seating arrangement, so was I now separated by my new physical difference. Back in the hospital, all of us patients had ostomies, and it was the typical thing in that place. But here in the real world, I was an oddity. My friends could never really understand what it was like to have an ileostomy – to be constantly checking for leaks, as I discretely did now, and to be tethered to one's home because of those frequent leaks. They could never know what it was like to have such cleanliness issues and to suffer from skin breakdown around the stoma. I had made an appointment with Paulette for a Reiki session, but felt compelled to cancel it; it was just too far to travel to Long Branch and to risk leakage there or along the way. And so, I felt myself sinking into a deep depression; the emotional pain which now encompassed me was more profound and more intense than all the physical pain which I had thus far endured.

But this depression also gave me an insight into the human condition. It was this: physical pain, because it was bound up in one's finite body, does have its limits, although they may be far off. But the depth of emotional pain, which is seated in the intangible psyche, can be boundless. And so, after having completed my OT psycho-social fieldwork more than two years earlier, I finally developed an appreciation of what the clinically depressed patient must suffer.

And had it not been for the action which I then took, I too would have become clinically depressed. That Sunday evening I called Claire, Debbie's mom. Claire had an ileostomy since she was eighteen.

"It's a mechanical problem, which you will resolve in time," she counseled. "At first, it's expected that you'll have leakages." And then she told me about the products which she used for her ileostomy.

"What brand bag and wafer are you using?" she asked.

I told her. The hospital had given me several boxes of supplies.

"I know what you have. It's the transparent bag. You should order the beige bags. You don't have to be looking at that stuff."

Claire highly recommended that I consult with the ostomy nurse who had helped her control her own leakage problems many years back. I took down her telephone number.

"I'm also going to contact an ostomy support group. They meet in New Brunswick," I told Claire.

"That's okay for now," she said, "but don't let the ileostomy become the main focus of your life. It's not, and it doesn't have to be. But that's what may happen if you join a support group. You can have a full life with an ileostomy. I got married and had children. I go out with friends. It doesn't stop me from doing anything that I want to do."

Of course, I also called Dr. Stark, to fill him in on how I was doing. He told me that had I not gone to the gym to prepare for the surgery, I would surely be in rehab right then.

My next step was to contact the head of the support group, who gave me loads of practical advice over the phone. And then I called the home health care agency to which the hospital had referred me, and made an appointment for an ostomy nurse to come to my home later that week to evaluate my stoma and the products I was currently using for it. Debbie Z, the nurse, showed me how to care for the sensitive skin around the ileostomy, and she showed me products which would conform to the particular contours of that skin. These materials would act like a washer to keep any feces from leaking out from under the wafer. Then I ordered these items through a surgical supply company. It would take a few more weeks for me to perfect their application; several times, I was woken up in the middle of the night by a tickling sensation under my wafer, and it always turned out to be the beginning of a slow leak.

Although after this adjustment period I would still be plagued by leaks from time to time, my brief glimpse into clinical depression had thankfully come to a quick end. Nevertheless, I felt different from others. About twice each week, in the morning, I now had my routine of putting on a fresh wafer and bag, on a completely empty stomach, after I had showered. I'd have all my supplies ready on the bed. But Mike, who was often still home at that hour, would avert his eyes from the stoma. It was ugly, I knew, and even he must have found it painful to gaze at. When I was dressed, you'd never know that I had this physical difference from other people. Unlike others who had gone through bodily alterations because of illness or accidents, I was able to conceal this ugly aspect of my physicality. To those who were not aware, I appeared normal. I was so fortunate.

Nearly two weeks after returning home, I was still on antibiotics for my urinary tract infection, and, as advised by Dr. Wong, I made an appointment to see a urologist. In order to urinate, I had to bear down hard on my abdominals, and normal, full bladder sensations were still missing. Memorial Sloan Kettering only had one urologist, and I didn't want to travel to Manhattan, so I arranged to see a local doctor. Gary left work early to drive me to the urologist's office in a nearby town. The doctor catheterized me and removed about 200 cc's of residual urine from my bladder.

"Well, you've been to hell and back," he said flatly. "You're very lucky to be able to urinate at all. Sometimes normal bladder functioning never returns after such extensive abdominal surgery. I want you to catheterize yourself daily for the next two weeks to measure any residual urine in your bladder after you urinate."

A large amount of residual urine would put me at risk for recurrent bladder infections, and I would then have to catheterize myself daily for the rest of my life. I was quite bummed out at that prospect, but as I've learned to do, I "re-framed" my situation. This I did by simply telling myself, "Thank G-d I'm not a man!" It helped tremendously. But Debbie Z told me that I risked infection by catheterizing myself. So, I simply used all the force which my abdominal muscles would allow, and bore down hard to try to completely empty my bladder each time I'd go to the bathroom. And then I threw away the catheters.

Our health insurance company sent us a letter, stating that they would not pay for the last week of my hospital stay. Little did they realize that, although I was in pain and still very dizzy, I had plenty of time at my disposal, and was fully capable of composing scathing letters to them. I recruited the help of a patient advocate at Memorial Sloan Kettering, who provided the company with documentation to prove that my extended hospitalization was necessary. After several months and a decision by an independent review board, the insurance company agreed to pay all but the last two days of my hospital stay.

Paulette had told me that the post-operative pain was just "residuals." I had quite a lot of those. Besides the sore, inflamed skin around my stoma, my lower back still ached, as did my abdomen, and I frequently felt a sharp, knife-like pain in the upper part of my scar. The right upper quadrant of my abdomen was aching dully, which made me wonder if Dr. Fong had possibly removed part of my diaphragm along with the liver tumor. My left leg also hurt. After giving birth to Lia, I developed varicose veins and had a localized phlebitis there. Since then, whenever I wasn't feeling well, my leg would ache. It was like a barometer to alert me that something was not right. Well, I didn't need a barometer to tell me that, because every afternoon, I was now running a slight fever. On top of all this, now that I was post-radical hysterectomy, my hot flashes came on with a vengeance and much more frequently than before the surgery.

To help myself get through this recovery period, I went back to Internet joke sites; I spent several hours each day searching for good jokes which would give me a belly laugh. And with effort, I began to slowly read books again.

Mike had been doing the shopping, and my neighbors were always stopping by to see if we needed anything from the supermarket. Lia had been my laundry helper, lifting clothes in and out of the washing machine and then helping me to sort through them, with me sitting on my bed to conserve energy. And Rhonda had insisted on giving me the gift of having her cleaning lady come over for a day to clean the house from top to bottom. Gradually, I began to cook again, and, seeing that I was becoming more functional, my mother stopped coming over in the mornings to "baby sit" me.

Finally, I was permitted to drive, which I did, despite still feeling quite dizzy. If I simply focused on the scenes outside of my windshield and didn't turn my head too quickly, I was able to travel to familiar places. And one of those familiar places where I longed to go was Long Branch – to Paulette.

Making the trip down the shore was another milestone in my recovery. In case I should spring a leak, I brought a knapsack filled with ileostomy supplies. Whenever I traveled a long distance or was planning to stay away from home for several hours I would take this along.

The appointment was for late morning, for Paulette had said she wanted me to sleep as long as possible and rest.

"It's like you've come back from a war," she noted, as I entered her apartment.

The subtle scent of lavender, spice, and musk once again greeted me, and I slowly inhaled it, trying to hold it forever in my lungs. Cellular memory.

"I feel like I've returned from one. All wounded."

I walked over to the spare room which housed the Reiki table. Paulette had thoughtfully placed a small stepstool beside it so that I didn't have to strain myself to climb up. I then sat down and lowered myself onto my back by walking my elbows backward.

"You did that very well," said Paulette with a smile. She gazed down at me on the table. "Talk to me."

How fortunate I was! For there stood Paulette, with her gentle but direct and non-judgmental manner of relating to people – me among them.

"What would you like me to talk about?"

"About how you're doing. How you're feeling. Perhaps your thoughts."

I told her all about my aches and pains, the fever which I had been running in the afternoons, and the unresolved dizziness.

"How did you ever manage to drive here?"

"I managed. I can do it."

Then closing my eyes, I put my hands at the top of my abdomen, over the most painful part. Paulette turned on the familiar music, which brought a broad smile to my face.

"Perhaps at this time," she said, "you should be thinking about what you are supposed to be learning from your experience."

I nodded as she placed her warm hands upon my head. The lessons which we are supposed to learn, I was quite sure, are multifaceted. One of the lessons, I was certain, was to trust in G-d and in his goodness. This has been one of the most difficult lessons for me to learn, especially as there are so many horrible things happening to so many good people. But there were other lessons, as well.

"I think," I told her, after some thought, "that pain is a tremendous catalyst. Why G-d uses this as a way to teach us, I'll never know. It's a rather old-fashioned method, don't you think?"

Paulette chuckled. "I suppose it is."

"Old-fashioned, but effective. You see, I think I always had compassion for other people. But that feeling was something very abstract inside my head, perhaps because I myself had never really suffered. But now, after what I've been through, whenever I hear that someone is in a lot of pain, I can close my eyes and practically feel what it is *they* feel."

"You've grown up," said Paulette in her gentle way. "Now I want you to focus on feeling gratitude. Thank you, G-d."

We suspended our conversation, and she continued the Reiki in silence.

The things which I had learned were nothing new to the world. Nearly 2,500 years ago, Aeschylus, the Greek playwright, had worded it much better than I ever could:

> He who learns must suffer. And even in our sleep, pain that cannot forget falls drop by drop upon the heart. And in our own despair, against our will, comes wisdom to us, by the awful grace of G-d.

That's not to say that I was now infused with wisdom. But perhaps I had a bit more insight into the suffering of others.

And then, happily for me as I lay on the Reiki table, I once again felt embraced by that Great Presence as I focused my mind on the gratitude which I felt for having successfully come through my own painful ordeal.

"Your symptoms are not unusual, and they will resolve over time," said Dr. Wong, after Dr. Ojibwe had removed the stitches from my former mediport site. We were at my post-op visit. He reiterated that the margins around the tumors had all been clean.

"But, just as a precaution, you'll have to go on follow-up chemo. Dr. Ilson will be in touch with you to set up the protocol."

After having been through five cycles of chemo in the spring, I had great respect for the havoc which it can wreck upon one's body. Somehow, I would have to gear myself up mentally to go through it again.

Slowly, my residual symptoms began to dissolve. It was only my bladder sensations which never quite returned to normal. But I was still functional as far as that went.

It was time for my post-op appointment with Dr. Salwitz. He told me that Dr. Ilson, who was out of the country for the time being, had contacted him regarding my follow-up chemo, and that he wished to discuss it with me.

"Dr. Ilson feels that you don't need to have the follow-up chemo."

My heart leaped from joy. Yes! I was done with it all! Yet, my mind wouldn't let me rest until I knew the rationale behind Dr. Ilson's decision.

"Dr. Ilson says," answered Salwitz, "that there have been no studies done on the effectiveness of follow-up chemo on people who have had stage four colorectal cancer."

I listened closely. This didn't sound like a very good rationale at all.

"But," he continued, "there are only about 2,000 of you in the country, so of course, no studies have been done on such a relatively small group, and no studies will ever be done. However, you had seven viable lymph nodes." That could mean that there were still some cancer cells in me.

"So why," I asked, "does Ilson not want me to have the chemo? It sounds like a no-brainer to me."

"He's just going strictly by the book. I consulted with one of my colleagues about Ilson's opinion, and we said, 'Nah, that can't be right.'"

I sat on the examination table, soaking in everything Dr. Salwitz said. As Dr. Soffin, the radiologist, was to later tell me, "The problem with Memorial Sloan Kettering is that they don't think outside the box."

"They took out my mediport in the hospital. Would I have to get another one put in?"

"Nope. We can do it intravenously."

I was liking this more and more. "Talk to me now about the chemo."

"It'll be nothing like what you had before," explained Dr. Salwitz. "It's going to be a very low dosage, administered for only five consecutive days one time each month for four months. And instead of having to sit in the clinic for three hours, it'll take only fifteen minutes to administer it to you. There'll be virtually no side effects."

His energy and exuberance were getting me charged up. This was going to be an unexpected walk in the park.

"What about the fatigue factor?" I asked. I had to know everything.

"There won't *be* any."

Now you can fully appreciate the value of having a Dr. Salwitz, in addition to the doctors of Memorial Sloan Kettering. He offered a different, independent perspective and, in this case, the more sensible one. In my mind, I started to formulate a new visualization: The Terminator and I would go house to house, cell to cell, and hunt down and destroy, with flame throwers and machine gun fire, every last, lurking, ugly, little cancer cell in my body.

"So," Dr. Salwitz finished, "what do you think?"

My mind had been far away, off on a preview of the next crazed, murderous rampage on which I would soon mentally embark. I looked at him, and was brought back to reality.

"Let's do it," I said.

The Open Door

The blood work which I had taken at my post-op visit to Dr. Salwitz showed that my CEA level was now 3.0. Almost normal! So near, yet so far! Mike and I were very excited about it. I was tantalized by the number 2.5 – which was now just within reach. It marked the threshold between cancer and health. How I longed to cross that border!

It was now two months after my surgery, and my symptoms, except for an occasional stabbing pain at my upper scar, had amazingly all resolved. I was back at the gym, on the elliptical, going easily on level two, for I still babied my abdomen. It would take me months to build up again to level ten, and then several more months to surpass that and have level twelve as my gold standard.

Bob caught sight of me as I pedaled along. He started to wave his arms and jump up and down like a kid. I couldn't help but smile from ear to ear.

"Wait!" He called from across the gym. "Don't go anywhere!"

Of course I wasn't going anywhere. There was an hour of cardio for me to get in.

Bob jogged over to me as I continued to pedal the foot plates.

"How are you feeling? I've been speaking to Mike, and he's been filling me in on everything."

I told him about the follow-up chemo, which I was scheduled to begin the coming week.

"You'll breeze right through it. Just continue what you've been doing. So tell me," he continued, changing his focus, "what did you do before your surgery, after I told you to pull back?"

"Oh, Mike and I went hiking in Holmdel Park."

"Hmm. I find the trail maps there to be confusing."

"Yes they are," I answered. "But I like getting lost and then finding my way."

Bob smiled. "That could be a metaphor for your life."

Yes it could. But in my case, I had several key people – Mike chiefly among them – who guided me along.

The follow-up chemo started out uneventfully, without any symptoms. So that I would not have to keep getting re-stuck with a needle, I asked the nurses to leave the butterfly IV in my forearm, taped down, for a few days at a time. I even went off to the gym like that. When the tape loosened there, I went to the front desk and got some scotch tape to hold the needle in place. But before the end of the first cycle, I started to get a slight sore throat. By the weekend, not only was my sore throat severe, but I had painful sores inside my mouth and on my lips. By Sunday evening, my lips and cheeks were very swollen, and it was even difficult to talk. Swallowing any solid food – even my vitamins – was impossible. It felt like shards of glass going down my throat. And it was excruciating to swallow my own saliva. Because my lips were so tender and swollen, I couldn't even hold a cup or a glass to my mouth. I was able, though, to slowly sip chicken soup or tea through a straw. Brushing my teeth was sheer agony. On top of this, I started running a fever in the afternoons. But worst of all, to my dismay, the skin on my chin developed dark blotches. My skin had always been my one good physical attribute.

"It's all from the chemo," explained Angela, one of the nurse practitioners in Salwitz's office. I had come in because of these extreme symptoms. She had the lab do some blood work on me then and there. My white blood cell count was normal.

"If it were low, we'd have to hospitalize you."

"I'm not going back to any hospital," I answered determinedly.

She prescribed an antibiotic and an oral pain elixir.

"It's very important that you keep drinking – you mustn't let yourself get dehydrated. We can give you IV fluids now in the clinic to keep you hydrated. We'll find you an empty chair."

That's one of the last things I wanted – another IV.

"No thanks. I'll go home and hydrate myself through a straw."

I dared not go to the gym, for there it was necessary for me to continually drink water as I sweated on the elliptical. The way I was now, I wouldn't be able to drink fast enough to keep from getting dehydrated.

"Stop the chemo!" Mike begged me. He couldn't bear to see me suffer.

"No way! I want to live!" I insisted, my swollen tongue making me stumble over my words.

No way would I give up now, after having come so far. The end of the tunnel was practically in sight.

Fully recovered from the surgery, I was now hungry, but unable to eat. Totally miserable, I daydreamed about sinking my teeth into a nice fat bagel smothered with cream cheese and stuffed with lox. When this was over, I told myself, I'd go out and buy myself that bagel. And I'd get it with real, high-fat cream cheese, which was not allowed on my anti-cancer diet. But I'd allow myself this one treat as a reward.

Mike had been suggesting ever since I returned home from the hospital that we revisit Dr. Simone. We actually did go to him before I began the follow-up chemo, and at that time Dr. Simone increased my dosages of his vitamins and nutritional supplement. Now, after my first cycle of follow-up chemo, we returned to him.

"I'm surprised that you can even sip warm drinks. Usually, people with mouth sores like yours find it more soothing to drink cold liquids," said Dr. Simone.

He then advised me on what to do.

"You're going to love this. Have you ever eaten raw eggs?"

"I hate eggs of any kind."

"I was afraid you'd say that. You can use egg substitute, then. I want you to get a gallon of ice cream. Whole ice cream. I'm not concerned about the fat content, because right now, you need the calories. Now what flavor 'Super Energy' are you using?" That was his powdered supplement which you add to water.

"Orange."

"Try the vanilla," he said. "That seems to work best with ice cream. Do you have a blender?"

"Yes."

"Good. I want you to put three large scoops of ice cream into a blender, and add to that two scoops of the 'Super Energy.' Then add either two raw eggs or the equivalent in egg substitute. Then, take the vitamins (i.e., Dr. Simone's vitamin, mineral, and amino acid supplements) and pulverize them. Just put the pills between two pieces of waxed paper and crush them with a hammer. Add this to the ice cream and eggs, and mix it up in the blender. This will give you complete nutrition for the day, and it will feel cool and soothing going down. Also, instead of drinking water during the day, I want you to either drink juice, skim milk, or broth. Everything that goes into you must have nutritional value."

Then I described to Dr. Simone the agony of brushing my teeth.

"Here's what you do," he said. "Get some hydrogen peroxide. Make a mixture of half hydrogen peroxide and half water. Dip your toothbrush into this mixture and use it instead of toothpaste. It'll disinfect your mouth but will be gentler than using toothpaste. And don't use mouthwash! That contains alcohol, which will be very irritating to you. If you find that the peroxide mixture is too strong, you can weaken it a bit by simply adding more water."

Dr. Simone's advice was a G-d send, and it helped me to get through the mouth sore episodes, which lasted about a week and a half and were repeated each month that I had the follow-up chemo. During those periods, I couldn't drink juice of any kind, as he had suggested, because it was too acidic, but cold milk was tolerable.

Dr. Simone's advice once again pointed out to me the importance of having several, independent resources; not everybody has the same knowledge base – no one person is a complete encyclopedia of help and information. And, it is a well known fact that most doctors know very little about nutrition – it's a subject that isn't stressed in medical school. You need a professional, preferably an MD who has delved into this area, in order to have proper guidance.

After I told Dr. Salwitz about my extreme symptoms, he reduced the potency of the chemo; otherwise the sores would have gotten worse after each cycle, and I would have had to be hospitalized with IV fluids.

My hair began to get extremely thin. In the mirror, my head resembled a baby bird's, with uneven tufts of sparse downy feathers. So that my partial baldness would be less glaring, I had my hair cropped very short. Although I didn't loose my eyebrows or lashes, my armpit and leg hair fell out. When I told Lia about this, she gave me her teenage perspective: "You're so lucky!"

Fortunately for me, Mike and I had those tickets for a Broadway show which we had ordered back in the summer. We saw *Spamalot*. Mike found it tolerable, but I enjoyed it tremendously, for it had just the right amount of camp and obscenity to keep me laughing. For a few hours, I was able to completely forget my pain. We also made plans to go away to a hotel in the Catskills with Risa and Allen, Rhonda and Elliot, and some other people for the weekend of New Year's Eve. That, too would give me yet something else to look forward to as I got through these chemo cycles.

Each month, I saw Dr. Salwitz for my exams and blood work. At the beginning of December – December 4 to be exact – I had an appointment with him. Could I delay the next chemo cycle for one week, I asked him, so that the side effects wouldn't interfere with our planned trip?

"No problem."

"Talk to me now about remission," I said. For months, Lia and Zack had been asking me when I would be in remission. I promised that I would speak to Salwitz about it at this visit.

Dr. Salwitz went over to the laptop on the counter. He printed out a small graph.

"This represents your CEA levels over the months. They've been going down steadily, but they really plummeted after your surgery. Right now, your CEA level is 2.3. Normal, as you know, is between 0 and 2.5. Remission means no evidence of disease. You have no evidence of disease. You are in remission. Congratulations."

His words left me stunned. They were everything I had longed to hear. He was now giving me full credit for this achievement.

"But it wasn't me who did it," I stammered. "It was G-d."

Dr. Salwitz gave a slight nod of acknowledgment. "Yes, it was G-d, but he gave you the tools and you used them. You used them very well." He then shook my hand in a vise-like grip. "You are healthy and vital. *And* beautiful. Congratulations."

In a daze, I left his office, my heart beating wildly as the significance of this news took hold of me. It was as if a dungeon door had swung open for me to step out into the light. Remission – the most beautiful word in the English language. Remission. I had been set free.

"So," I thought as I walked to my car, "this is what it's like to be reborn." It was a bright, balmy day for December, unseasonably warm. The late afternoon sun infused the sky with a golden glow and lit the way home. The excitement in me grew as I anticipated telling Mike the incredible news. As I drove along the curving road which led to the highway, a welling sensation rose inside my chest – a sensation which grew until it felt as if I would come apart at the seams. There just wasn't enough room inside me. I was not large enough to contain all that I felt, for now my heart was bursting with profound gratitude.

Mike surprised me one day, after my first mouth sore episode had nearly completely cleared up, with that bagel and lox sandwich of which I had been dreaming. Relishing each bite, I chewed it slowly and carefully because, as Dr. Balsh had warned, large chunks of food in my intestine could cause an abdominal blockage in my ileostomy. Always, I made sure to chew my food completely.

So, it was strange when I woke up in the middle of a Friday night, late in December, with what felt like intense gas pains. My ileostomy bag was filled with gas and nothing else. The pain was nagging, and I tossed and turned, unable to get back to sleep.

That morning, I had no appetite and felt very bloated.

"I think I'm getting an abdominal blockage," I told Mike. Then I tried massaging my stomach, and lay supine on the floor with my knees raised to my chest, as suggested in some information materials we had gotten from the local ileostomy support group. Nothing worked.

"Maybe we should go to the hospital," suggested Mike, worried.

"Let's see if it'll clear up." Despite the pain, I was in no hurry to be a hospital patient again.

But the pain only got worse. It was different from the post-surgical pain. That pain had been steady. This pain came in intensifying waves, and I felt it from my abdomen through to my back. A feeling of nausea grew in me, and I went to the bathroom to vomit.

"That's it. I'm taking you to Robert Wood Johnson," declared Mike. "Call Dr. Salwitz."

I began to cry. "I don't want to be a patient again!" I knew I was being irrational.

"Ruth, we've got to go. Look at you."

I was doubled over in agony. Succumbing to the pain, I called Dr. Salwitz's office. He was away on vacation, but one of his associates, Dr. Reid, was on duty. He told me that it sounded like I had a blockage and to get over to the hospital emergency room immediately.

It seemed to take forever as I lay on the gurney in the emergency room. I was taken for an x-ray and then, after slowly drinking the contrast fluid, a CAT scan. Afterward, I told the nurse that I felt nauseous. He handed me a small kidney-shaped dish.

"I need a bucket."

As soon as he gave me the larger basin, I vomited what appeared to be all of the pink contrast fluid. I was still in agony.

An emergency room resident came to our curtained cubicle. "The CAT scan shows that you have a partial abdominal blockage. We'll soon have a bed for you. I want to give you something for the pain. Have you ever had Percocet?"

Back in Memorial Sloan Kettering, I had once vomited shortly after being given Percocet. I didn't want to risk having a bad reaction.

"Percocet makes me hurl."

"We could give you morphine."

That sounded good to me. A nurse injected a vial of morphine into my vein through an IV which had been inserted into my arm.

I felt my heart speed up and my blood vessels suddenly constrict, as if my entire body were put inside a vise. Then, the pressure sensation eased up and there was a feeling of release. A pleasant drowsiness took hold of me, and my pain completely vanished.

Mike went with me as I was wheeled to a private room in a hospital ward filled exclusively with patients from Dr. Salwitz's oncology group.

Another resident on duty, a young woman in green scrubs, came to my bedside.

"I'm going to have to put an NG tube in you. It's going to empty out your stomach contents."

So, the NG tube had finally caught up with me. There was no getting away from it.

"When are you going to put it in?" I asked.

"Now," she answered decisively.

"I'd like to brush my teeth first."

"All right. I'll come back in an hour. And I'm also going to put a Foley catheter in you."

"No you're not." I didn't want to get another urinary tract infection. Nor did I want to go through another episode of not being able to urinate after the catheter was removed. "I'm able to get off the bed and go to the bathroom."

"We need a way to measure your urine output," she said authoritatively.

Wiser now, after my experience at Memorial Sloan Kettering, I answered her, "Put a hat in the toilet."

"And how are you going to get to the bathroom when you're hooked up to the NG tube?"

"I'll *un*hook it." You could unhook the tubing from the pump. "It's not rocket science."

The doctor looked annoyed and left the room in a huff. So what? Let her stew. I needed to protect myself from their overzealous medical management.

As promised, the resident returned about an hour later and stuck the NG tube down my nose and throat. It was horrible, and it made my throat feel very sore. I wasn't allowed to eat, and I certainly didn't want to, but I was given a pitcher of ice chips to suck on. However, I was so thirsty that I developed the strategy of letting the ice chips melt and then drinking the cold water. Toward evening, I settled into the hospital bed and dozed off from the morphine.

In the morning, after unhooking the NG tubing from the pump on the wall behind me, I went to the bathroom, brushed my teeth, showered, and dressed. The ileostomy bag was absolutely empty. My stomach contents were not moving through my intestines at all, but were being slowly sucked out through the tube. I tried walking around the halls, but after five minutes had to return to my room because of the stomach pain. After rehooking the NG tube, I lay down on the bed. Before too long, a nurse asked me if I wanted more morphine. Definitely. Again, I felt the terrible tightening sensation, and then the release. I tried to focus my eyes to read a bit.

"Mrs. Levine?"

Somebody was repeating my name over and over again. As if called back from far away, I opened my eyes to find two men, one in green scrubs and a lab coat, and the other in a cable sweater, standing at the foot of my bed.

The one in the sweater introduced himself as Dr. August. The other guy must have been his fellow.

"I'd like to examine your abdomen."

Dr. August palpated my stomach, which caused quite a bit of pain.

"You have a partial abdominal blockage around the site of your ileostomy. This often happens after having had abdominal surgery. What happens is that the intestines can twist up around the scar tissue. You've had very extensive surgery and have a great deal of scar tissue. Usually, the NG tube relieves the pressure on the intestines by emptying out the stomach contents, and the blockage clears up."

"What happens if it doesn't clear up?"

"Then you'll need surgery to remove the scar tissue and clear up the blockage." An intestinal blockage, he explained, is a life threatening situation, as the twisted intestines can become gangrenous. "And there's no guarantee that you won't have another blockage in the future."

G-d, no. I couldn't bear the thought of going through another painful recovery. And, Dr. Wong didn't operate out of this hospital.

"Who would operate on me?" I asked.

"I will," said Dr. August.

I didn't know who the hell he was. It was time for a brief interview.

"Have you ever done this kind of surgery before?"

"Yes," he answered.

"How many of this type of surgery do you do a week?"

"About five."

All right. He was probably very experienced. Now I wanted to know more about how I would be affected.

"Where would you cut me?" I asked

"Probably right where your scar is."

"And how long an incision will you have to make?" The bigger the incision, the more painful the recovery, of course.

"That would depend. I can't give you any guarantees."

I would have to pray that the NG tube did its job.

Dr. August fished his hand in his pocket.

"Here's my business card. Hopefully, you won't need any surgery. We want to empty your stomach contents completely. So, you can't even drink water. Just suck on ice chips to wet your mouth."

I told Dr. August about my previous strategy of letting the chips melt.

"You're not the first patient to come up with that idea." And then he stressed the importance of limiting my liquid intake.

Then he and his fellow left. I looked at the business card which he had handed me. It said:

David A. August, MD., P.A.C.S.

Professor of Surgery

Chief, Division of Surgical Oncology

UMDNJ-Robert Wood Johnson Medical School

Did he ever get grilled by any other patients, I wondered, as if he were a novice? Oh, well, better safe than sorry.

Later that morning, Mike came by with my mother and Gary. Unfortunately, I had an episode of severe nausea and vomiting, followed by dry heaves. Being from the "old school," my mother had a hard time understanding how I could possibly get better without eating. Surely there was some food which would cure me! The head of my bed was elevated, as this position reduced the feeling of nausea. Surely it would be more restful for me to lie flat! I began to get aggravated at her well meaning but potentially harmful meddling. After I had been given another dose of morphine and became very drowsy, they got up to leave. My mother whispered to Mike to lower the head of my bed. I heard that.

"Leave it alone!" I snapped.

They didn't touch the bed controls, but let me doze off into my morphine-induced state of nirvana. It came on effortlessly with the dosage I was given. What I felt was similar to the effects of Reiki, but without all the concentration and visualization. So, I realized, this was why drugs were so appealing!

"I have a surprise for you," said Mike over the cell phone the next evening. I was already dressed in hospital gowns, ready for bed. I wondered what the surprise could be and begged him to tell me.

"You're going to have a visitor in a little while."

"Who?"

"You'll see."

It was Debbie and her husband, Mitchell. They were returning after dropping off their younger son at the airport. It was Christmas break, and he was going to Florida to spend some time with his grandparents. After saying hello and asking how I was, Mitchell left the room to let us talk.

Debbie looked down at the meager contours of my body under the blanket.

"Before you know it," she said, "you'll have shrunk down to nothing."

"I'll soon be looking like you," I told her. Debbie was very petite.

Debbie looked very concerned. "Are you in a lot of pain?"

"It's starting to come on again, but it's nothing like when it first started. I'll soon ask for another shot of morphine before I'm ready to go to sleep."

We chitchatted about small things, and Debbie told me all about her son David's trip. But I could see the concern in her eyes. I began to perspire profusely.

"Are you all right?" she asked.

"It's just a hot flash. It'll pass."

Debbie got a washcloth, wrung it out in a bit of ice water, and put it on my forehead. It helped a lot.

"Are you able to get out of bed?"

"Of course. I try to walk around in the halls every day, but I can't do too much with the pain. I've gone on their computer, though. They have a computer with Internet access in the lobby outside the room. Mike went on the Robert Wood Johnson website and saw that they're looking for an occupational therapist. He says I should apply while I'm here."

The congested commute to Robert Wood Johnson didn't exactly thrill me, but who knew? Perhaps it was such a good place to work that it would make even that worthwhile.

"Are you going to do that?" asked Debbie.

"Why not? An interview will at least be good practice, even if I don't get hired. I asked Mike to bring all my credentials and a copy of my resumé. I'll stop into Personnel and drop everything off."

Debbie laughed. "I can just see you marching down to the Personnel Office in your hospital gown and handing them your resumé. You *would* do that, too."

"Well," I said, "their Personnel Office is in another building, so I'll at least have to put on a coat."

The nurse came in and asked if I wanted another dosage of morphine. My stomach was starting to hurt badly.

"Let me go to the bathroom first and brush my teeth."

I disconnected the NG tube from the pump and shuffled over to the bathroom with the curved tube taped and hanging from my nose. It looked like I had a thin elephant's trunk protruding from one nostril. When I got back into bed, the nurse injected a vial of morphine into my IV. Once again, I felt the terrible, vise-like pressure in my heart and limbs, and then the slow release. I tried to keep my eyes open, but the pleasant drowsiness which spread through me was overwhelming.

· "I'm going to go now and let you sleep," said Debbie, smoothing the blankets around me. "I have no doubt they'll hire you – and they'll be happy to have you."

She bent over me to adjust the cool washcloth which she once again put on my forehead.

"And you're going to be a *good* occupational therapist," Debbie said quietly into my ear, "because now – after everything you've been through – now you know what it's like on the other side of the bed."

The Closure

I spent a total of five days in Robert Wood Johnson University Hospital and, fortunately, did not need surgery to clear up the blockage. My ileostomy began to function again, although my abdomen remained quite sore for some time from the entire episode. After listening for bowel sounds, Dr. Reid decided that I could go home. To play it safe, I kept myself on a bland, mostly clear liquid diet and used a juicer to extract the pulp from any fruit that I ate. Unfortunately, Mike and I had to cancel our trip to the Catskills, which seemed to disappoint Risa more than anybody. The rich hotel food would have been intolerable for me.

"Can't you come and just not eat?" she had asked over the phone.

Her request was too absurd for me to get angry.

As soon as we returned home from the hospital, the telephone rang. It was the personnel director of Robert Wood. She wanted to set up an interview for me with the director of rehab.

The interview suit, which had fit so perfectly at the beginning of August, now hung from my frame. Not having had the time to take it back for alterations, I took up the slack in the waist with a safety pin.

I felt self-conscious about my hair.

"Do I look hideous?" I asked Mike, certain that I did.

Mike looked me over. "Your hair is just a little thin, and if someone really thought about it, they'd realize that you've had chemo. But you don't look hideous. To me, you're always beautiful."

And more importantly, I was healthy. As Bob had happily proclaimed, after I had told him that I was in remission, "Fuck the hair!"

Still uncertain whether I looked odd to everyone else, I drove off to my interview.

I didn't think it had gone very well. You could see from my resume that I was a new graduate. Nevertheless, the director, dressed in a formal pink suit, asked me, "What are your clinical skills?"

Well, damn, I didn't have any clinical skills. All I had was my knowledge of what it means to be a patient.

"That is not a clinical skill."

Surprisingly enough, about a week later, I got a call from the personnel director, offering me a per diem position at the hospital. Boy, they must really be desperate for a real, live OT, I thought. But I declined their offer, because I had already found another job.

It was near my home. I had answered a magazine ad. Over the telephone, the regional rehab director, who did the hiring, asked me what I had been doing since I had graduated. I told her. At the interview shortly afterward, she didn't even bother to ask about my "clinical skills."

"I know that you have no clinical skills," laughed Toni. "But you have a lot of life experience."

She got that one right.

And so, with one more cycle of follow-up chemo to go, toting along my ileostomy supply knapsack each day, I began to work five half-days a week. Mostly, I was doing evaluations of new patients. Occasionally, I would come across a patient who was similar to me. One of them was an older woman who had a new colostomy, after having been diagnosed with colon cancer. It was obvious to me that she was still depressed and stunned by what had been done to her.

"You're pretty strong, physically, for someone your age," I told her. "You're going to make a great recovery."

But she only sat at the side of her bed and stared with hopeless eyes.

"Look," I continued. "There's something I want to show you."

Then I lifted my scrubs shirt and pulled away my pants a bit to reveal my own ileostomy bag.

"See, I have an ileostomy. It's similar to a colostomy. You'd never know it. I'm able to do anything that I want to do. I work. I go to the gym. I do everything."

Her eyes widened. "Will you look at that!" she wondered in amazement.

It was my hope that she too would come to terms with her physical alteration and go on with her life. She had great potential.

Although the dark blotches on my chin had happily cleared up, I was now starting to experience neuropathy in my hands. It became very difficult for me to do fine motor tasks such as buttoning and engaging the zipper of my jacket. My new colleagues would sometimes joke with me in the therapy gym, announcing, "The OT needs OT!" Dr. Salwitz had reassured me that this too would resolve after I was done with the chemo.

From time to time I would still experience the beginning of an abdominal blockage, but, fortunately, I discovered that one way to resolve it was with lots of moist heat. Whenever I felt a blockage coming on at home, I immersed myself in a very warm bath, getting out every so often to force myself to vomit. This took the pressure off my stomach and helped my intestines to relax. Only once did Mike and I have to revisit the emergency room for a blockage which I couldn't fix at home.

As I neared the end of my follow-up chemo cycles, I was filled with mixed feelings. I was happy that I would no longer experience those horrible mouth sores – during which period I still had to drink Dr. Simone's nutritional concoction in lieu of eating solid food. But the chemo had become a psychological crutch. As long as I was undergoing treatment, I knew that I could keep the cancer at bay. Once it ended, I would be flying solo.

"A lot of people feel that way," said Dr. Salwitz, when I expressed those concerns to him. "Don't worry. We're going to keep you on a very short leash."

Part of that short leash consisted of having monthly blood work, in addition to CAT scans every four months. I now was due for one, plus another visit to Dr. Wong, in mid-February.

Apprehensive as I was about approaching the end of the follow-up chemo, I told Paulette how I felt.

"Perhaps you should come up with a new affirmation," she suggested. "Something positive to remind yourself that you are now healthy."

After some thought, I came up with this one: I am watched over and sheltered by a *loving* G-d. To me, this summarized my feeling that I was under the wing of an actively mindful Higher Power, without there being any guarantees of being totally protected.

Sometimes during Reiki, as I cleared my head of the "chatter" which constantly went on inside it, I would come to various insights.

"You know," I told Paulette, "back when I was doing my Level II physical disabilities fieldwork, I couldn't bear to see a patient's amputated limb. It was just too painful for me to look at. And I certainly couldn't identify with anyone who had that done to them."

I was thinking specifically of a patient at work with a below-the-knee amputation. Earlier that week I had helped him don his gel-sock stump covering and his prosthesis as well.

"But now that I have this ileostomy," I continued, "these things don't bother me any more. I know what it's like now to have your body altered. Now I'm one of *them*. It's as if the barriers have come down."

"You've learned a great deal from your experience," said Paulette.

I nodded. Then I told her about my Reiki session back in the summer with Karla, when she had me visualize in detail about myself.

"I just realized," I continued, "that everything I visualized has come to pass exactly as I saw it."

"Yes," said Paulette. "*All* things are possible. You have indeed come a long way in a very short time. Be *very* grateful for where you are today."

I definitely was. Then I quieted down and focused on the light energy which surely flowed through her hands. And that light, which I had first envisioned a year earlier as a thin, slowly meandering stream of clear molasses, had now become a rushing river.

"Have you heard about Dr. Stark?"

Debbie had called me, and I hadn't any idea what she was talking about.

"What do you mean?"

She then hesitated. "I wasn't sure if you knew."

"Knew what? Tell me." I wasn't going to let her get off the phone without telling me all.

Debbie sighed. "I thought you probably knew. I'm sorry now that I brought it up." She paused. "He has cancer."

It was like a punch in the solar plexus.

"Ruth, are you alright?"

I was breathing heavily. "Uh huh."

"He has a lot of patients, you know, and word gets around. I heard that he collapsed at a conference at a hospital and that they did some tests on him then and there. They found out that he has melanoma and it metastasized to his brain."

It felt like I was being diagnosed all over again, except this time instead of feeling panicky I was overcome with a blanket of sadness. Dr. Stark had been one of the foundation blocks in my moral support system. Who could have known that while he was bolstering me, cancer was quietly growing within him?

I called Dr. Stark's office, but the receptionist, because of privacy laws, couldn't give me any information or updates. Have him call me, I asked. He did that evening.

"I'm feeling fine and have already begun treatment," he said, his words slightly slurred. "I fully expect to be back in the office in six months."

He sounded totally positive and had me believing this expectation.

To help Dr. Stark get through this tough period, I wanted to give him something. But what? He had such a positive attitude to begin with. And I wasn't a physician who had the power to change or enhance his outlook with medicinal words. So I told him how Reiki had helped me and said that I would forward information on it to him along with Paulette's telephone number, through his office.

Dr. Stark said nothing, but the silence told me that he probably would not pursue that path.

"I'll be thinking of you every day, Dr. Stark. And I will pray for you."

He thanked me, but I was one of his many patients, and I got the feeling that he preferred not to involve us too closely in his personal life. The relationship between a physician and his patient is not exactly reciprocal.

Then I told myself that I would make an appointment to have a checkup with him in the fall, and at that time we could both greet each other as fellow survivors.

"Your CAT scan shows some shading on the liver," said Dr. Wong at my office visit to him. "It could just be fluid, but we have to make sure. I want you to make an appointment to see Dr. Fong. He may want to order a liver biopsy."

I felt well, but naturally Mike and I were very concerned. When we got home, I called Dr. Salwitz.

"Why don't we just order a PET scan?" he said. "That will tell us if there's anything malignant."

Once again, Dr. Salwitz's clear, common sense, outsider perspective came shining through for me.

To be on the safe side, we took the films and report of the PET scan to Dr. Fong, who pronounced me healthy.

"There's no need for you to make any more appointments with me," he said happily. "Your oncologist in New Jersey is taking very good care of you. But if you like, you can send me a Christmas card every year to let me know how you're doing."

"I'll do that, gladly," I said. "For the next fifty years."

Going through a health crisis can help you put everything else into clear perspective. About a day or so after our visit to Dr. Fong, we came home to find a note in our door saying that there was a certified letter waiting for us in the post office. On my way home from work the next day, I stopped by to sign for the envelope and opened it up at the counter. After thoroughly reading the letter, which was from a lawyer, I burst out laughing. One of our crazy neighbors was suing us. He claimed that one of our cats had entered his home, had peed all over his living room carpet and stairs, and had damaged the top of his vertical window blinds. Mike and I both had a good laugh over this, as did our lawyer, who suggested that we simply have our home insurance company handle the claim. Rather than go to the expense of hiring our lawyer and perhaps having a Pyrrhic victory, this is just what we did. After all we'd been through, we certainly didn't worry about this little episode, but put it where it clearly belonged – on the back burner of absurdity.

I had opted to have my ileostomy reversal done in the summer, nearly a year after the original surgery. I could have had it done earlier in April, but I didn't want a painful recovery period to interfere with my preparations for Passover. Furthermore, Mike would not be working in the summer, and it would be easier for him then to make trips into the city to Memorial Sloan Kettering. Naturally, I was still going to the gym, and did not have to make a Herculean effort to prepare for this procedure.

About three weeks before the scheduled surgery, we had an appointment with Dr. Wong to sign the consent form, followed by pre-op testing.

"How big an incision will you have to make?" I asked him.

"About two or three inches long," he said.

I gave a wide smile. That was practically nothing.

Dr. Wong then explained about what would follow. "You're going to have an open wound after the surgery, and it'll take a few weeks for it to close up. The dressing will have to be changed daily. We can arrange for a nurse to come to your home and do that, or you can learn, while you're in the hospital, to do it yourself."

Well, it hadn't been a problem to change the wafer. Certainly, I could learn to change a dressing. "I'll learn how to do it myself," I said.

Dr. Wong told me that this operation would only take about two and a half hours. Could it be done, I asked, without a breathing tube or a Foley catheter inserted into me?

"I think so. You won't be under anesthesia for that long."

After I happily signed the consent form, Mike and I went on to the EKG, which this time was normal, and for the routine blood work.

To be honest, I wasn't exactly eager to go through another recovery from yet another incision, as small as it might be. But more so,

I was very concerned about whether my bowels would ever function normally again after my colon was reattached. So, although the ileostomy closure sounded like a fairly simple procedure and I knew that I would once again look normal after it was done, I still wasn't sure if I'd be functional. At least now, with the ileostomy, my bowels functioned after a fashion. And as long as the ugly piece of my exposed intestine was covered up, as long as it was hidden from view, nobody could know that I was in any way different – except for Mike. However, in that regard, Paulette had this illuminating comment: "Imagine what it'll be like when you have nothing there but *skin*."

But all that became a moot point when I got a call from Dr. Wong's nurse, who told me that there was a "slight" abnormality in my blood work. My CEA level was 6.0.

I was distraught. Was the cancer creeping back? We had planned to go away to Canada before the surgery to visit my cousin Susan, whom I hadn't seen in years, but if things were taking a turn for the worse, not only this trip, but the surgery itself would be put on hold. Dr. Wong would not close the ileostomy if I had a recurrence of colon cancer. But more importantly, my precious gift of good health would be rescinded. And it had only been the previous month, at my last visit with Dr. Salwitz, when I had mentioned to him that if I ever had cancer again, I knew I could overcome it. I should have kept my mouth shut, for our omniscient Lord, who hears all, seems to have an ironic sense of humor. Now I was back on the emotional cancer roller coaster.

Mike, although very concerned, tried to keep it all in perspective.

"Ruth, it's 6.0, not sixty. It's still in the single digits."

Try though I did to see things as he professed to, I was flooded with a sense of grief and loss. And I had worked so hard to get where I was and to stay there! Now G-d was simply pulling my chain.

At Reiki I told Paulette the latest news.

"I've done everything in my power to stay well," I said forlornly. "I go to the gym and work out like an animal. I'm very careful about what I eat, and I take all of Dr. Simone's supplements. I don't know what else to do."

Paulette wondered if perhaps there was some mistake with the test.

"I'll go to Dr. Salwitz and have him do his own CEA test," I said dispiritedly.

As I lay on the Reiki table, Paulette placed her warm hands on the crown of my head.

"Now take a few gentle breaths and focus on this light which is coming from G-d," she suggested.

During the entire time that I was ill, I had been accepting of G-d's will. Never had I been angry at him. But now, after having reached the crest of the hill of recovery only to be struck down to try to stagger upward again, I became tearful – and enraged.

"G-d can take his light," I hissed, "and stick it you-know-where!"

Paulette sucked in her breath, shocked at my sacrilege.

"You're angry!" Then, after a pause, she continued, "How about if you just see it as energy entering into you?"

Okay, I could envision energy as a neutral force, not as a vindictive or a capricious one. I closed my eyes, took a series of deep breaths, and tried to settle my feelings of grief and anger. Paulette started by placing her hands on the crown of my head, but after a while, moved to my side, put one of her hands over the spot where my liver was, and placed my right hand on top of hers. Mine kept slipping off, and she kept replacing it. Finally, to keep my hand from falling off, Paulette sandwiched it between her two hands.

Slowly, imperceptibly, I began to be filled with a profound sense of calm, as if I were beyond all the turmoil which was tearing at me. Somehow, I was being enwrapped in a safe, warm cocoon. How does she do that, I wondered.

Dr. Salwitz told me to come in immediately for a CEA test in his lab. It took one nerve-wracking day for the blood work to be processed. I was at work in the therapy gym when Dr. Salwitz called me on my cell phone with the results. My hands trembled as I opened the phone. He got right to the point: 1.6. Memorial Sloan Kettering had erred.

I still had the ileostomy closure done with Memorial, though. Mike and I didn't hold this little screw-up against them. I like to take the best of each resource. What I don't like, I simply discard. And Dr. Wong is one of the top colorectal surgeons in the tri-state area. If you should ever need his expertise – and I hope you never do – I highly recommend him.

My nurse said that I was a first. When I was brought to my room after being in post-op, I walked for twenty minutes with her beside me. I would have walked longer, but she couldn't let me do that alone immediately after surgery and she had to get back to work. The pain and dizziness were only a fraction of what they had been with the first surgery. And I was fortunate, because slowly, gingerly, after about two days, my bowels began to function.

The only bad thing about this second hospital stay was the coffee. It was horrible. Ever since I had begun to work, I needed two cups of brewed coffee every morning to wake me up. Now was no different. The coffee which they served with breakfast was instant. Dressed in my street clothes, of course, I headed for the elevators.

"Is everything all right?" asked one of the nurse practitioners, as I waited at the elevator bank.

"Uh huh. Be back."

The elevator opened, and I stepped in. With ten dollars in my pocket, I was headed for the Dunkin' Donuts on First Avenue. I needed some *real* coffee.

The elevator opened at a middle floor. In the hallway, lying on a gurney, was a man, somewhat younger than myself, with his head bandaged. He had obviously had recent brain surgery. G-d. Our eyes locked. As the elevator door began to close, I winked at him. Hang in there. And as if responding in silent code, he winked back. I will.

Then I thought of Dr. Stark. It would soon be six months since he had been diagnosed. I'd have to call his office to find out if he were back at work. I still prayed for him daily.

The night before I was to be discharged, I went for my evening walk in the halls. Now I had an MP3 player filled with all my favorite music. I went foraging in the supply closet: no hospital socks. At bedtime, I liked to wear a fresh pair of non-skid socks in the hospital, so that if I got up to go to the bathroom, I wouldn't have to go fishing around for my slippers. You'd think they were more valuable than plasma, the way they rationed them. I went over to the nurses' station.

"Can I have a pair of hospital socks?" I asked the receptionist.

She looked at me, dressed in my street clothes.

"Are you a patient?"

That word! How I hated to be called that! It was so insulting – a term of enfeeblement and powerlessness. I bristled.

"I'm not a patient! Don't call me that!"

The receptionist glanced at the hospital bracelet on my wrist.

"Oh," she smiled knowingly, "then what are you?"

I bent my face close to the window slot. With a lowered voice, and in my most serious tone, I answered her confidentially.

"I'm a prisoner of war."

The receptionist smiled. "Go back to your room, Mrs. Levine. I'll have someone bring you a pair shortly."